HEALTH EDUCATION
MADE EASY

HEALTH EDUCATION MADE EASY

Dr Robert Peprah-Gyamfi

Perseverance Books
A Division of Thank You Jesus Books
Loughborough, Leicestershire, UK

HEALTH EDUCATION MADE EASY
Copyright © 2012 Robert Peprah-Gyamfi

Published by Perseverance Books
A Division of Thank You Jesus Books

For information, please contact:
THANK YOU JESUS BOOKS
P.O. BOX 8505
LOUGHBOROUGH
LE11 9BZ
UK

ISBN: 978-0-9570780-3-1

www.thankyoujesusbooks.com

Acknowledgements

⟨~⟩

M y heartfelt thanks go to God Almighty, Creator of heaven and earth, for imparting the wisdom needed to write this book; Rita, my wife, together with our children Karen, David, and Jonathan, also deserve my thanks and appreciation for their support and encouragement, which enabled me to persevere to the successful conclusion of this work. I am also grateful to Dr Charles Muller of Diadem Books.com for carrying out the editorial work and for writing the Foreword.

TABLE OF CONTENTS

FOREWORD

⌒

T HIS IS a health education manual with a difference! First, it
is clearly written, in a friendly and easy to follow manner that
will make it invaluable for the layman who does not have a full
understanding of how the human body functions, to come to grips
with the essential causes of diseases and medical cures. The writer,
himself a medical doctor, often writes from the perspective of his
own early background in a rural village in Ghana, and, indeed, for
anyone growing up in an African context, this book will be a won-
derful guide to better health. The analogies the writer uses make it
so much clearer for the reader to grasp the functions of the body.

The *Manual* is very readable, all the more so on account of the frequent illustrations from the doctor-author's own consulting room.
There is the woman, for instance, who comes to him complaining of
night sweats and unaccountable swings of mood. In the traditional
African context she and others might have thought that the sudden
and inexplicable condition pointed to witchcraft. Similarly, the
sudden inexplicable death of a successful businessman who appeared
to be robust and healthy might have made Africans brought up in a
traditional context suspect, again, the wiles of a witch doctor. The
author, however, shows how both of these instances are explained
by established medical science—the onset of menopause, in the case
of the woman, and high blood pressure, which is often undetected,
in the case of the businessman.

The *Manual* is consistent in its logical and methodical structure, where each condition or complaint is explained through a systematic pattern of health risks that might trigger the disease or condition (like breast cancer), causes of the condition (like genetics—it might be an established pattern in the family history), symptoms of the condition or disease, methods of diagnosis (like clinical examination), and principles and methods of treatment or cure.

It is a practical book, and an informative one, too, for if the reader has had any lapse or gap in his or her education or schooling in biology and physiology, this book will bring the reader up to speed in a friendly and even entertaining manner, for this doctor knows how to sweeten the pill! With his attractive bedside manner, he speaks to the reader not as a superior doctor but as a friend and as an equal, never pedantic and never aloof.

As a health manual, this book is especially helpful. Very readable and even entertaining on account of the friendly narrative style and the telling illustrations and examples, it can be read for general information and education about the human body and its functions; but perhaps more important, it can be used as a reference book, to be consulted on specific health issues when such health issues become relevant, perhaps to put the reader's mind at rest or possibly confirm the appearance of a medical condition, such as breast or prostate cancer. Either way, the book is a good companion, to keep in the bookshelf, on the coffee table, or by one's bedside!

Charles H. Muller
Diadem Books
MA (Wales), PhD (London), D.Litt (UOFS), D.Ed (SA)

PART 1

PREVENTION IS BETTER THAN CURE

CHAPTER 1

He Who is Not Sick Needs No Physician

PREVENTION is better than cure—that is a well-known saying. For example, instead of treating a patient with full blown clinical symptoms of cholera, it is better in the first place to provide the individual with clean drinking water, clean sanitation and also to educate the individual about the need to maintain good personal hygiene.

He who is not sick needs no physician. Let us pause a moment and consider our world suddenly transformed into a world free of disease—yes, a world populated only by healthy individuals. Imagine that—a world of healthy people where there is no diabetes, no arthritis, no HIV, no malaria, no mental illness, no cancer! Arguably, the number of the unemployed would suddenly shoot up into the high heavens resulting in possible social unrest as all our hospitals, policlinics, health centres and psychiatric institutions closed their doors and sent their entire staff home for lack of work!

If indeed prevention is better than cure, there is the need for each and every one of us as individuals to do whatever we can to prevent disease.

This brings to mind what I learnt from my driving school teacher in the northern German city of Hanover several years ago. He taught his driving class that three factors come into play the moment a driver joins the flow of traffic. These are:

1) The driving skills of the individual involved.
2) The condition of the vehicle he or she is driving.
3) The other drivers on the road, the condition of the road and the elements.

Whereas one can influence the first two factors, our teacher pointed out, the individual is completely at a loss as to the third factor. He urged us always to do all we could do to minimise the chances of becoming involved in a road traffic accident by positively influencing the first two factors. For example, we should never drive under the influence of alcohol or when we are too tired, or too unwell to do so.

Concerning the second factor, he advised us always to make sure the vehicle we are driving is in perfect condition—with properly functioning brakes, good tyres, well-functioning lighting systems, etc.

In a sense, that thinking can also apply to the area of our health. It is said that the best defence is attack. In the area of medicine, I will modify that saying to this: the best cure is prevention! So let us make this our highest priority—the prevention of disease.

CHAPTER 2

Some Paths to Disease Prevention

THERE ARE several methods of disease prevention. These include maintaining good personal hygiene, drinking clean water, assuming a healthy lifestyle eating a balanced diet, exercising regularly, not smoking, avoiding alcohol completely or drinking it moderately, exercising on a regular basis, avoiding stress, etc.

KEEPING FIT THROUGH EXERCISE

There is indeed a general consensus among health care professionals concerning the beneficial effect of regular physical exercise to our health. Apart from preventing us from becoming overweight or obese, regular exercise can indeed help protect us from several diseases. These include heart disease, stroke, high blood pressure, Type 2 diabetes, obesity, back pain, and osteoporosis (a disease in which the bones become extremely porous and are subject to break or fracture). For some, exercise even helps to improve their mood.

There is clearly, therefore, a need for us to exercise our body on a regular basis. The question that arises is: how much exercise is enough? There is no clear-cut answer to the question. I will call for a common-sense approach.

Much us we are called upon not to overeat, I think when it comes to exercise it is also important that we do not overdo it, that we do not do more than our body can cope with.

For example, if you have been inactive for a while it is better to start with less strenuous activities such as walking or swimming at a comfortable pace. Beginning at a slow pace will allow you to become physically fit without straining your body. Once you are in better shape, you can gradually do more strenuous activities.

Most experts agree that moderate exercise for 30 minutes every other day is adequate to help improve the cardiovascular function, to lose weight, reduce stress as well as lower cholesterol and blood pressure.

STRESS AVOIDANCE

We should not lead an idle life, not sit down doing nothing and hope that manna will fall from heaven to feed us. Still, it is important that we guard against overstraining or overworking ourselves. It could among other things, lead to what the doctors call Burn-Out Syndrome (defined as chronic work-related stress) which in turn could adversely affect our immune system.

I have heard the story of some citizens from my native Ghana resident in London who leave home in the morning to work eight hours at Workplace A, move on from there to Workplace B to do another six hours of work only to move to Workplace C to do another four hours of work.

Some hardly make it back home to have a shower before moving back to start another day's work at Workplace A. Where do they keep and change their clothing? Well, the story goes that some keep their toiletries in their bags. They have their showers at their places of work! As far as food is concerned, they either carry it along or purchase some from one of the numerous fast food chains around. And what about sleep? Well, according to the story, they do so during their travels on public transport—the Underground and the London buses. Some are said to fall so deep asleep during their journeys that they miss their stations and are usually awakened at the end station by the station assistants during their routine checks on the trains.

The body of the individual I referred to may perhaps be able to cope with that degree of stress for a while. One does not need to have a degree in medical science or be a prophet, to predict that should that strain on the body continue for a while, it will sooner, rather than later lead to the breakdown of the individual involved. We are mortal human beings after all, we are not machines. And even machines need periods of respite for maintenance and repair. The body can cope with stress over short periods, but stress, when it becomes chronic, can adversely affect our health and lead to the following: weakening of the immune system, headache, upset stomach, stomach ulcer, high blood pressure, heart attack, etc.

CHAPTER 3

Breastfeeding as a Way of Disease Prevention

THOUGH it may not be obvious to everyone, breastfeeding is a means of disease prevention, for breast milk, apart from providing the means of energy and growth for the new-born, also provides needed antibodies to boost the immune system of the new-born. As far as possible, therefore, effort should be undertaken by mothers to breastfeed their babies for a minimum of six months .

You and I are aware that today, industry has come up with formula milk. Now I am not saying that this is not a good thing. As in all instances of our existence, industry, once it has come up with a product, will go to great lengths to sort of push the product onto the consumer.

Agreed, there are instances when mothers are unable to breastfeed on health grounds. I should like at this stage to recall my childhood in my little village in Ghana. I remember at the time when I was growing up there when mainly as a result of disease a new mother was not able to breastfeed her baby, other women, those already nursing their babies, stepped in to help out. In some instances, some women who were even not breastfeeding at that time took over that function. Somehow the body registered the need to produce milk in the extraordinary circumstance and began producing milk!

Due to the factors outlined below, it is recommended that, as far as possible, new mothers undertake efforts to breastfeed their babies for a minimum of six months .

Protection against infection and diseases. As I mentioned above, breast milk is rich in antibodies. These are passed on to the child. This leads to a strengthening of the body's defence force. This helps to protect against some of the infections common in the early stage of life.

Antibodies passed from a nursing mother to her baby can help lower the occurrence of many conditions, including:

- ear infections
- diarrhoea
- respiratory infections
- meningitis

It has been established that breast-fed infants are less prone to diseases as compared to infants who receive formula.

Mothers living in a place like my little village Mpintimpi will tell you, usually during the time when they are breastfeeding their children, the children usually look well-nourished and also less susceptible to infections.

The problem begins during the transition to normal feeding and thereafter. Soon they not only begin to display signs of malnutrition, they also become susceptible to infections.

Besides protecting against infections, the strengthening of the immune system can protect the baby against allergies which in turn could minimise the risk of developing asthma.

Nutrition and ease of digestion. As I mentioned earlier, the body requires carbohydrates, fat and protein to grow. All the three components are present in breast milk. The good thing for the baby is that they are present in a form that makes it easy for the new-born's immature digestive system to absorb them.

It's Free. Breast milk doesn't cost anything, so it is affordable to even the poorest mother walking the earth's surface. The author of these lines really does wonder what would have happened to him if his impoverished parents were forced to resort to formula milk to feed him!

Different tastes. It has been established that breast milk has different flavours depending on the meals eaten by the mother. Breastfed babies are thus introduced to different tastes through their mothers' breast milk.

Ease of Availability. It's available whenever and wherever the baby needs to be fed. Mothers who breastfeed are thus spared the last-minute dashes to the store for more formula as well as the need to warm up bottles, sometimes in the middle of the night.

Breastfeeding mothers are able to actively go about their activities with their babies, knowing that they'll have food available whenever their little one is hungry.

Obesity prevention. Some studies have found that breastfeeding may help prevent obesity.

Skin-to-skin. The skin-to-skin contact between mother and child in breastfeeding can enhance the emotional connection between mother and infant.

Breastfeeding does not only facilitate the health of the baby, but that of the mother as well. Breastfeeding helps burn the calories of the mother and helps shrink the uterus, so nursing mothers are able to return to their pre-pregnancy shape and weight a lot sooner than those who resort to formula.

Studies have also shown that breastfeeding helps lower the risk of contracting cancer of the breast, the ovary and the womb.

PART 2

TERMINOLOGY DEFINED

Before I tackle some of the most common diseases around, I shall spend some time to explain some of the common terminologies that may confront us not only in this book, but in our day-to-day involvement with issues relating to our health. These are:

- The Immune System
- Infection
- Fever
- Balanced Diet
- Ideal Weight
- Cholesterol, Good and Bad

CHAPTER 4

The Immune System

W E ARE surrounded by billions of bacteria and viruses poised at penetrating our body to cause us harm. Our skin forms a thick wall which prevents this from happening.

In addition, the skin also produces a variety of substances that are harmful to potential invaders. Openings such as the eyes, nose, and mouth are protected by fluids or mucus, a slimy substance that capture harmful attackers. The respiratory tract also has mechanical defences in the form of cilia, tiny hairs that remove particles. Intruders that get as far as the stomach are usually destroyed by stomach acid.

In spite of the above outlined defence mechanisms, hostile invaders still manage to get through. Some enter along with our food, while others may do so through the nose. Cuts or scrapes to our skin also provide avenues of invasion for the micro-organisms. The immune system helps protect us from the micro-organism poised at invading the body to cause harm to it.

The defensive cells, also known as immune cells, are part of a highly effective defence force called the immune system. The cells of the immune system work together with different proteins to seek out and destroy anything foreign or dangerous that enters our body. It takes some time for the immune cells to be activated – but once they're operating at full strength, there are very few hostile organisms that stand a chance.

Immune cells are white blood cells produced in large quantities in the bone marrow. There are a wide variety of immune cells, each with its own strengths and weaknesses. Some seek out and devour invading organisms, while others destroy infected or mutated body cells. Yet another type has the ability to release special proteins called antibodies that mark intruders for destruction by other cells.

Our immune system is not only intelligent; it is complex and at the same time sophisticated. I do not want to delve into further details in the matter. Those interested to know more are advised to source the relevant literature on the topic. What we have to know is that we can through our attitude, diet, lifestyle, etc., either strengthen or weaken the defensive capabilities of our formidable army.

CHAPTER 5

Infection

INFECTION is a term we all encounter on a regular basis. What does it mean?

As I mentioned in the previous chapter there are billions of microorganisms—bacteria, viruses, yeast, fungi, etc., constantly attempting to invade our body system.

Diseases brought about by such micro-organisms are classified as infectious diseases. The list of infectious diseases is long. They range from the common cold to the potentially life-threatening diseases like cholera, malaria, meningitis, etc.

Infectious diseases can be passed on from one person to another. There are several avenues by which this can happen:

- Droplets: Infectious organisms may be passed on by means of droplets containing them. This can happen through sneezing, coughing, talking, etc.
- Ingestion: This can be achieved through eating contaminated food or drinking contaminated water.
- Sexual contact: Several kinds of infection can be sexually transmitted.
- Skin: Infectious organisms can penetrate the body following injury to the skin.

CHAPTER 6

On the Meaning of Fever

WHEN I worked as a family doctor in Dusseldorf in Germany, the majority of my patients were from Ghana. On not a few occasions some of them came to the consulting room with the words, "Doc, please help me—I have fever." In most instances the temperature of the patient turned out to be normal. Thereupon, I made it clear to the patient that he or she had no fever.

"But I feel feverish, Doc. I really do believe I have fever!"

It is indeed important for a doctor to understand the cultural background of the patients he or she is dealing with to properly understand their needs! Whereas a patient from Ghana will tell you "I have fever" when he/she wants to let you know he/she feels generally unwell, an English patient will tell you he/she is "feeling poorly". Indeed, prior to my arrival in the UK it never occurred to me that a person who was vomiting would describe that condition as *"I am being sick."*

This leads me to the term *fever* as it is applied in medicine. To help us maintain a stable milieu within our body system in the presence of ever-changing environmental conditions, our body is imbued with several self-regulatory mechanisms. This is particularly important, since our body was created to function within an almost constant body temperature range of between 36.5–37.5 °C (98–100 °F).

How do they do so on a planet that can be as hot as the Sahara and as cold as the Arctic?

Well, the hypothalamus, an area in our brain, is assigned the responsibility of maintaining a normal temperature range as stated above. The hypothalamus is responsible not only for the maintenance of a constant body temperature but several other regulatory functions in the body. The hypothalamus achieves this goal with the help of agents known as thermoreceptors located in several parts of the body.

Disease, in particular, infectious disease, can disturb this control mechanism and lead to a rise in body temperature above the set norm. A fever can be caused by many different conditions ranging from benign to potentially serious.

Moderate rises in body temperature do not usually require treatment, for the body is capable of coping with such rises. Whatever the cause of fever, the moment it rises beyond a certain point, especially in children, there is a need to take steps to help bring it down. Though the underlying cause may not cause problems, the very fact that the temperature has risen above a certain level could lead to problems including what is known as febrile convulsion.

This takes me back again to my childhood days. Malaria was and is still endemic in Ghana. I remember in not rare instances, little children whose bodies had turned "hot", as we put it, who would suddenly begin to have a fit. Lay people as we were in the matters of medicine, we at that juncture instinctively began to pour cold water on the affected child. In many instances that led to an improvement of the condition. We did not really understand the mechanism involved. Naturally we were delighted at the favourable outcome of our action. If only we had known that the rising temperature could lead to the fit, we would have administered paracetamol (if indeed it was available) earlier on to avert the situation.

CHAPTER 7

Balanced Diet

$\backsim$

I WILL USE an example from my own life in an attempt to shed some light on the term balanced diet. When I was growing up in my little village in Ghana, we usually had for breakfast and also lunch a meal prepared from boiled plantains or yams, or cocoyams and kontomire (leaves from the cocoyam plant).

The main meal for the day was the evening meal, *fufu*. *Fufu* is made by pounding boiled cassava, plantain, yam or cocoyam into balls and swallowing small portions of the ball with soup. Meat or fish or both are added to the soup, though for our family meat and fish was a scarce commodity. The larger part of the little meat and fish we could afford was reserved for the adults, especially father.

We did not eat fruit on a daily basis. We had some oranges, peas and bananas, and pineapples growing on our farms—but we enjoyed them only during their seasons.

On the whole, the quantity of food I was privileged to enjoy every day was adequate. Indeed, none of us at home needed to starve. Still, *much as I tried* to grow tall, I did not grow taller than 165cm.

Now my son David is 15 years old as I write. At that age he has already passed the 170cm mark and is growing taller and taller. It is generally believed that the height an individual attains is dependent on the individual's parents as well as environmental factors. Now as far as the parent factor is concerned, though I am not a tall man, I am nevertheless taller than Rita, my wife. So we can rule out the genetic factor as the cause of David's increasing height.

This brings me back to the issue of a balanced diet. The various types of foodstuffs at our disposal need to be eaten in the right proportion to have an optimal effect on our bodies.

As a child, I was fed mostly on carbohydrates. That provided me sufficient energy to allow me to go about my daily activities, including walking a total of four miles to and from school. Without sufficient supply of proteins, vitamins, mineral elements, etc., my body however could not grow optimally.

My son David on his part has been privileged to enjoy not only an abundant supply of the various kinds of foodstuffs needed by the body, but also in proportion favourable for optimal growth.

Having said this by way of introduction, I wish to explain the concept of a balanced diet as defined by the experts in that area of human endeavour.

As I mentioned above, our body needs various kinds of food items to grow. These are classified into the following groups: carbohydrates, fat, proteins, vitamins, mineral salts and fibres.

Carbohydrates provide the body with energy. Examples of food rich in carbohydrates are: rice, maize, wheat, yams, plantain, cocoyams, etc.

Proteins on their part are required for growth and repair. They are obtained from fish, meat, beans, etc.

Fat, like carbohydrates, is a source of energy. Some vitamins, known as fat-soluble vitamins, are able to dissolve only in fat.

Vitamins are required in small quantities. They are however invaluable to the body since they help bring about several important reactions that take place in our body. Vitamins can be obtained, among others, from fruit such as oranges, apples, bananas, strawberries, etc.

Minerals: Several types of minerals are needed by the body for optimal growth and function. Examples of minerals needed by the body are: iron, calcium, sodium and iodine.

Fibre: Also called roughage or bulk, fibre is necessary to promote the wave-like contractions that move food through the intestine. High fibre foods expand the inside walls of the colon, easing the passage of waste.

As fibre passes through the intestine undigested, it absorbs large amounts of water, resulting in a softer and bulkier stool. By helping to form a softer, larger stool, fibre thus helps prevent constipation.

Examples of foodstuffs rich in fibre are whole fresh fruits, green leafy vegetables, root vegetables, whole grains beans, etc.

A balanced diet is a diet which contains the above ingredients in the right proportions. As a general rule, such a diet should contain about sixty per cent carbohydrates, twenty per cent protein and twenty per cent fat.

Vitamins and minerals, though vital to the functioning of our body, on their part, are required in very small proportions.

Not only are we to eat a healthy and balanced diet, we must also resist the temptation to overfeed ourselves. The saying has it that "too much of anything is bad". When it comes to the food that we supply to our body, one might indeed agree with the above saying.

The body needs a certain amount of energy each day in order to function properly. This energy is expressed in calories. The number of calories in a food depends on the type of food involved. One gram of each of the three main types of food—carbohydrates, fat and proteins—provides 4, 9 and 4 calories of energy respectively.

The daily calorie requirement of an individual depends on age, height, weight, gender, and activity level. For example, a soldier who has to undergo strenuous exercises on an almost daily basis will require much more calories per day than someone like myself who spends much of his day working on the computer.

As a starting point a female adult with low activity levels requires on the average 2000 calories to maintain a desirable weight, whereas her male adult counterpart with a similar activity level requires about 2,700 calories per day for the same purpose.

People who consume more calories than they burn off in normal daily activity are more likely to be overweight. The reason is that the body converts the extra energy into fat for further storage.

We can indeed draw a parallel with money. In daily life, the majority of us struggle to make ends meet financially. Some, however, manage to obtain those pieces of paper and coins that have been produced by countries to serve as a medium of exchange in surplus—indeed, in some cases in real abundance. Instead of carrying the surplus bank notes and coins around in bags, cartons, suitcases, etc., they choose to deposit them in banks. Usually the banks are able to keep them safe, until perhaps the next credit crunch sets in to threaten them.

There is an important difference between the excess food we eat and the excess money we possess! Whereas we can deposit the excess money in the bank or donate it to charity, for purposes far away from our homes, we can neither deposit the extra fat built up in us outside our body nor donate some to an individual dying of starvation somewhere on our common planet. So in due course we become overweight! We can, as it were, afford to become a little overweight. Beyond a certain limit, however, the additional weight can lead to a horde of health problems. Among other things, it can increase our risk of developing diabetes, high blood pressure, cardiovascular (heart and circulatory) diseases, etc.

CHAPTER 8

Ideal Weight

O N THE ISSUE of an ideal weight, one may well ask the question: what then is an ideal weight? There is not a general consensus among the experts in the matter as to what exactly is the ideal weight of an individual. In this book, I will reproduce two of the common references in use.

Broca Index:
This index originated from Paul Broca, a French surgeon, in 1871. It calculates an ideal weight in terms of the height and weight of the individual.

The Broca Index defines an ideal weight as follows:
Ideal Weight (in kg) = Height (in cm) – 100, plus or minus 15% for women or 10% for men.

Following this formula, the ideal weight for Miss Eve, 160cm in height, would be between 52kg and 69kg. Mr Adam, boasting the same height as Miss Eve, on his part, would have an ideal weight between 54kg and 66kg.

BMI Index:
Others resort to the more complicated **BMI** or Body Mass index whereby a BMI is calculated based on the formula:
BMI = mass (kg) / height2 (m2) for the metric-system, or
BMI = mass (lb) × 703 / height2 (inches2) for the imperial.

Still using Miss Eve as an example: Assuming at a height of 160cm she is found to weigh 80kg, her BMI would be 80/(1.6 x1.6) = 31.25 and would be classified as obese.

BMI Interpretation
BMI 18.5 to 25 Normal or optimal weight
BMI > 25 Overweight
BMI < 18.5 Underweight
BMI < 17.5 Extremely underweight
BMI = 30 or BMI > 30 Obese
BMI = 40 or BMI > 40 Morbid obesity

You may perhaps wish to use the above formula to calculate your BMI and then determine whether you are, perhaps, heading towards the category 'morbid obese'.

I hasten to add that the above information is provided to educate, not to scare! I believe that with a certain degree of self-discipline, most of us would be in a position to maintain a reasonable weight.

Before I leave this field, I should like to give my personal opinion about anti-obesity medication, medication meant to help reduce weight. I must stress that the optimal method of weight reduction is through a healthy or proper diet and regular exercise.

In my opinion anti-obesity medication should be reserved for those who have health problems relating to their obesity, for example high blood pressure, diabetes, etc. It could also be used as an initial help for individuals very determined to lose weight through diet and exercise. They should be discontinued after a while, after they have served their initial purpose whilst the affected person maintains the habit of eating a healthy diet and engaging in regular exercise. That, however, is my personal view on the matter. One is free to accept or reject it.

My opinion is based on my experience in general practice. There have been instances in the past when some of my patients bent on reducing weight have requested me to prescribe them such medication. After the initial weight reduction, brought about not only by the medication, but also by their determination to maintain a healthy diet and engage in regular exercise, some came back a few weeks later to confess that while indeed the "soul was willing, the flesh was weak." That became evident after taking their respective weights. After the initial weight reduction in the few days following the beginning of the anti-obesity therapy, some had returned to their initial weights; some had even surpassed their pre-therapy weights.

Finally: it should be borne in mind that like almost every medication, anti-obesity drugs are not devoid of side effects.

CHAPTER 9

Cholesterol "good" and "bad"

THE WORD *cholesterol* has gained a negative connotation over the last few years due partly to reports about it in the media. What many may not know is that it is needed for building and regulating cells. In other words, cholesterol is necessary for the normal functioning of our bodies. There are actually two types of cholesterol, low density lipoprotein (LDL) cholesterol as well as high density lipoprotein (HDL) cholesterol.

The negative effect of cholesterol on the body relates to LDL and not HDL. It is indeed true that too much LDL cholesterol in the body can cause problems to the affected person. This can lead to part of the LDL settling on the walls of the blood vessels to build up what is termed "plagues". In time, the lumen or the inner open space of the affected vessel can become narrower and narrower. This could eventually lead to the blockage of the vessel concerned. If this happens to the arteries supplying the heart and the brain, it could lead to a heart attack or stroke respectively.

It is important to reduce the amount of cholesterol consumed. One way of achieving this is to limit the consumption of food rich in cholesterol such as eggs, milk, cheese and meat.

HDL Cholesterol, in contrast to LDL Cholesterol, is known to have a beneficial effect on the vessels, preventing them from developing "plagues". Consequently HDL Cholesterol is sometimes referred to as "good" cholesterol.

Some foods such as olives, olive oil, and most nuts and nut oils (also known as monounsaturated fats) as well as vegetable oils play a beneficial role in the body by increasing HDL while at the same time lowering LDL.

It must however be borne in mind that about 75% of the body cholesterol is produced in the liver; therefore our diet alone is not the all-deciding factor in the level of cholesterol in our body.

Some individuals are also born with a genetic disorder known as familial hypercholesterolemia. The body of the affected individual is not able to remove low density lipoprotein (LDL) cholesterol from the blood. This results in high levels of "bad" (LDL) cholesterol in the blood of the affected person. This in turn can lead to the following symptoms, even at a young age:

- Fatty skin deposits (xanthomas) over the elbows, knees, buttocks, the cornea (white part of the eye), etc.
- Deposits of cholesterol in the eyelids (xanthelasmas).
- Arteriosclerosis (narrowing of the arteries).

PART 3

COMMON MEDICAL CONDITIONS TREATED

As my German driving teacher taught us from the outset, when we are in traffic, there are certain factors that could affect us that we have no control over. The same applies to the matter of our health. No matter what preventive measures we adopt, we can still fall victim to disease. It is therefore important that we keep ourselves informed about some of the common diseases that afflict mankind. Understanding what causes them and the symptoms to look out for will enable us to recognise them, preferably in their early stages. Apart from primary prevention, early recognition and treatment forms another important aspect in the fight against disease. This is particularly true in the case of cancer. I will therefore turn my attention to some of the common conditions that afflict us. I will in most cases observe the following pattern:

1) Cause: I will explain the cause of disease based on the latest knowledge available to medical science.
2) Symptoms: I will highlight the common symptoms associated with the condition.
3) Risk factors.
4) Diagnosis.
5) Treatment: I will highlight the treatment possibilities.

CHAPTER 10

Headache

I **THINK** it is superfluous to attempt to define the term headache; everyone has in his or her lifetime experienced this condition. Medical science knows two types of headache.

- **Primary Headache:** This type of headache stands on its own. In other words it is not related to any kind of disease.
- **Secondary Headache:** This is the headache that happens when the patient is afflicted by another disease. For example, one of the symptoms of the common flu is a headache. In other words, the headache is secondary to the flu infection. Sometimes, however, a headache may be the symptom of a more serious condition or disease, such as a brain tumour or meningitis. Other examples of medical conditions that can lead to headache are high blood pressure, dental abscess, eye conditions, etc.

PRIMARY HEADACHE
Unlike the secondary headache, primary headaches are not caused by another disease or condition. The three common types of primary headache are: tension headache, migraine and cluster headaches.

- **Tension Headache:** Each and every one of us might have experienced a tension headache at one stage in our life. It is characterised by a dull, steady and achy pain on both sides of the head. The pain usually begins gradually and increases over a period of time. Tension headaches are associated with stress, anxiety and depression.

- **Migraine:** This is an intense, throbbing, pounding or pulsating pain that is often experienced on one side of the head. Victims of the disease usually report experiencing symptoms that serve as a harbinger or foreteller that announces the onset of their pain. These include visual disturbances such as light flashing before the eyes, a funny taste in the mouth or a strange smell.
- **Cluster Headaches:** These are a type of headache similar to migraine and sometimes described as agonising or excruciating by the affected person. Victims may also experience severe pain in the eye or temple on one side of the head as well as a watering of the eye and a runny nose. Cluster headaches may be triggered by certain kinds of drugs and also by alcohol.

DIAGNOSIS
- Taking the patient's history, including family history (it has been observed that some families are prone to headaches such as migraines).
- X-ray: Though it may not be useful in certain cases, in the case of a brain tumour, X-ray can be a helpful tool in the diagnosis.
- CT & MRI-Scan: These can help reveal several causes of secondary headache such as brain tumours, cysts, abscesses, aneurysm, etc.

THERAPY
At the time I was growing up in my little village, though we could not count ourselves with the most sophisticated of people, we were nevertheless aware that Paracetamol, Aspirin and APC (which stands for aspirin, paracetamol and codeine) could help relieve headache. So whenever any of us was afflicted with the condition, we made our way to one of the few petty traders in the village selling them (they were usually sold as single tablets!), bought a few, took them and hoped for a favourable outcome.

Indeed, common primary headaches respond well to the above-named medication. We should however guard against overusing them. Failure to do so could lead to a paradox situation in which the analgesics or painkillers that are supposed to cure our headaches themselves become their cause. Indeed, overuse of such tablets could themselves lead to headaches—rebound or analgesic headaches, as they are called.

CHAPTER 11

Anaemia

$\backsim$

THE TERM *anaemia* refers to the situation when there is less than the normal number of red blood cells or less than the normal quantity of haemoglobin in the blood. Haemoglobin is a pigment found in the red blood cell. It has the primary function of transporting oxygen from the lungs to the body tissues. Indeed, it is the pigment haemoglobin that gives red blood cells their characteristic red colour. When there is a shortage of either the red blood cells or haemoglobin or both, the capacity of the blood to transport oxygen round the body is decreased.

To understand the effect of anaemia to the body, it is important to understand the role blood plays in the body. These are the following:

1. It transports oxygen away from the lungs and around the body; and carbon dioxide from the cells back to the lungs to be breathed away.
2. It transports nutrients to the cells.
3. It carries waste products away from the cells to organs such as the kidney and liver for excretion from the body.
4. It helps the body maintain a constant temperature.
5. With the help of the white blood cells, it helps to defend the body from various organisms that invade the body to cause harm to it.

6. Blood also carries substances that help blood to clot in case of injury and in so doing helps prevent blood loss.

Blood has two components: the liquid part, also known as plasma, and the cells floating in it. Dissolved in the plasma are various substances including electrolytes, nutrients, vitamins, hormones, clotting factors, and infection-fighting antibodies. The cellular part of blood is about ninety-nine per cent red blood cells; the remaining one per cent is white blood cells.

The adult human body contains approximately five litres of blood; it makes up seven to eight per cent of a per son's body weight.

TYPES OF ANAEMIA

There are three main types of anaemia:

1) Anaemia caused by increased red cell destruction, for example sickle cell anaemia.
2) Anaemia caused by decreased red cell formation. This can result from the following: poor diet, diet deficiency in folic acid, iron and Vitamin B12; chronic disease such as HIV/Aids; Cancer, etc.
3) Anaemia resulting from blood loss: injury to the body, diseases that cause profuse bleeding and heavy menstrual bleeding could also lead to anaemia.

SIGNS AND SYMPTOMS OF ANAEMIA

These include the following:
1) Fatigue (feeling tired all the time)
2) Headache
3) Dizzy spells
4) Shortness of breadth
5) Palpitations (rapid and irregular heartbeat)

TREATMENT

Treatment of anaemia aims at correcting the underlying cause of the condition with the end goal of either increasing the number of red blood cells in the body or the amount of haemoglobin carried by the red blood cells, or both.

For example:
- Iron-Deficiency anaemia is treated with iron tablets or in some cases injections.
- Vitamin supplements may be taken to replace folic acid and vitamin B12 in people with poor eating habits.
- Some people suffer from what is known as pernicious anaemia. In such individuals, their digestive system is incapable of absorbing sufficient amounts of vitamin B12 in their meal. Such individuals are treated with monthly injections of vitamin B12.
- If anaemia is caused by chronic or severe disease, treatment of the underlying cause could lead to a normalisation of the condition.
- In certain instances, blood transfusion could become necessary to correct anaemia.

SICKLE CELL ANAEMIA

Before I leave the area of anaemia, I shall devote some lines to the condition known as sickle cell anaemia.

What does the term stand for?

Medical science refers to normal haemoglobin as HbA. Each individual is endowed with two copies of the haemoglobin gene. A completely healthy individual thus carries two HbAs—one from each parent.

People with sickle cell anaemia have a type of haemoglobin known as sickle haemoglobin (HbS), which is different from normal haemoglobin (HbA).

Those who have one HbA gene and one HbS gene are said to have sickle cell trait and are referred to as carriers. Those with sickle cell anaemia have two HbS genes

The red blood cells of a person suffering from full-blown sickle cell anaemia are destroyed faster than would be the case of the person carrying normal red blood cells. Sickle red blood cells have a lifespan of approximately ten to twenty days compared to that of normal cells, which is between eighty and one hundred and twenty days. The end result of the above situation is that the individual born with the condition has to live with chronic anaemia.

Normal red blood cells are smooth, round, and quite flexible. As a result they can bend and flex easily, and so travel around the blood vessels easily. Sickle cells on their part are stiff and sticky and as a result are not able to move easily through blood vessels. Furthermore, they tend to form clumps and get stuck in smaller blood vessels. This leads in the end to the blockage of the small blood vessels of the affected person which in turn leads to the disruption of blood circulation to the end organ.

SYMPTOMS

- **Sickle Cell Crisis:** Blockage of a blood vessel causes an attack known as a crisis. This is more likely to happen when the person is stressed by another illness, exhaustion, cold, dehydration, low oxygen levels (such as living in high altitudes or flying).
- **Organ Damage**: The intermittent disruption of blood flow brought about by blocked vessels can lead to damage of organs such as the liver, kidney, lungs, heart and spleen.
- **Chronic Pain:** The blockage of the vessels can also lead to severe recurring pain, especially in the bones.
- **Anaemia:** The constant breakdown of the red blood cells leads to anaemia.
- **Chronic Infection**: Sickle cell anaemia is also associated with recurring infections.

TREATMENT

There's no cure for sickle cell anaemia, but the frequency and severity of crises and their complications can be reduced by avoiding the triggers and prompt recognition and treatment of a crisis.
One can take measures to minimise the effect.

These include:
- Eating a good diet and taking supplements of folic acid, vitamin D and zinc.
- Avoiding smoking and alcohol (both of which can affect the condition of blood vessels).
- Vaccination against infections such as the flu, pneumococcus meningitis and Hepatitis B, etc. will all help reduce the risk of a crisis. Some patients are given long term antibiotics.
- Avoiding dehydration, cold temperatures as well as overexertion.
- In some instances, patients are given long term antibiotics.

TRANSMISSION OF SICKLE CELL

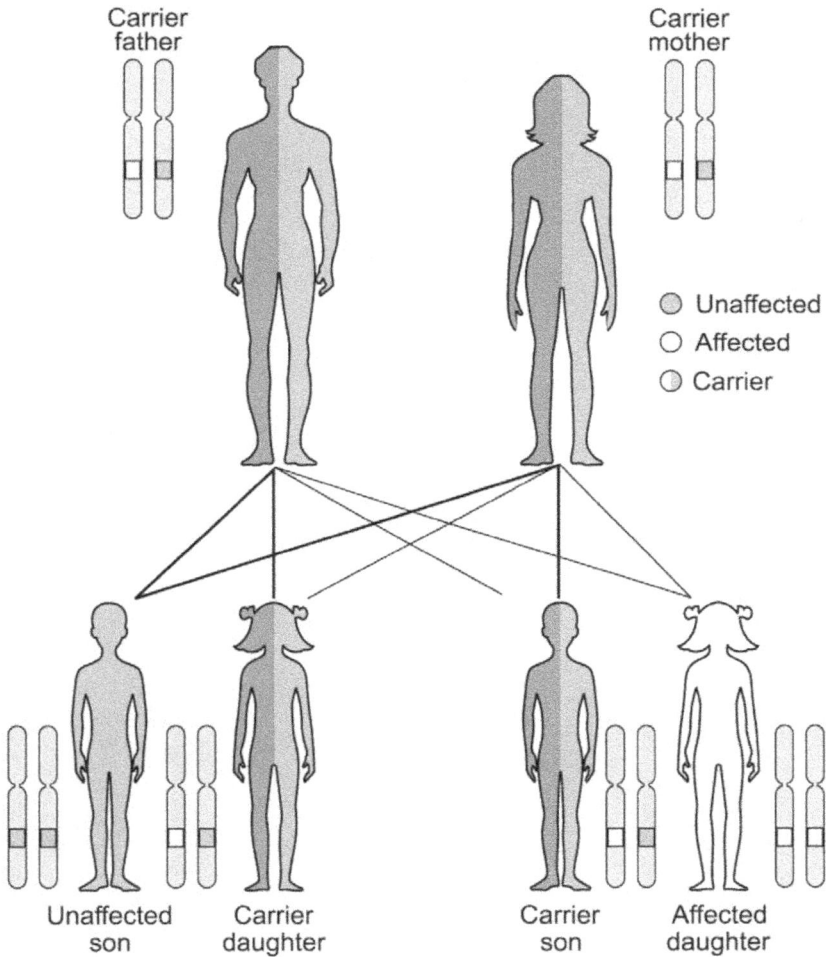

Illustration of how sickle cell is genetically transmitted

PREVENTION

Sickle cell anaemia can only occur when two people who carry the sickle cell trait have a child together. It is therefore advisable for an individual who is a carrier to avoid marrying another carrier of the disease… easier said than done! In the real world, who would go around testing the genetic constitution of a person he or she is attracted to before falling in love with such an individual?

CHAPTER 12

Hernia

W HEN I was growing up in my little village, there was a resident who had developed a hydrocele of the scrotum, a medical condition that leads to the accumulation of fluid in the scrotum. In the individual in question, the hydrocele had attained, without exaggeration, a really monstrous dimension. Those who are strange to the environment in which I grew up might ask: "Why didn't he seek medical attention?" The answer in short is poverty, poverty, poverty.

In the course of time word began to spread in the little settlement to the effect that one of the residents had been diagnosed with inguinal hernia. The doctors had recommended surgery. He had begged them to allow him to return to the village to gather the needed financial resources. Partly because he had in the meantime been feeling better, partly because he could not come up with the money required, he refused to return to the hospital. In the course of time someone told me that as much as the huge hydrocele of our co-resident was without doubt an embarrassment to him, it was not life threatening. On the other hand another resident afflicted with a hernia had a more dangerous condition that could kill him.

You may call it health education "Mpintimpi style". The doctors and other health professionals among us, those conversant with both conditions, will agree that my "health education instructor" was after all not entirely wrong in his assertion, for indeed a hernia can become life-threatening whereas a hydrocele of the scrotum rarely will.

WHAT IS HERNIA?

Our internal organs are wrapped in a transparent membrane (a plastic-like sac) called the peritoneum; this sack in turn is protected by the muscles of the stomach wall. The abdominal wall thus acts as a protective cover for our internal organs, in particular our intestines. In some instances, a tear occurs in the protecting wall. When this happens, parts of the internal organs, especially the intestines, bulge through the tear and appear as a lump under the skin. This is what is referred to as a hernia. Sometimes the weakness is already present in children, for example around the navel (umbilical hernia).

This again brings back memories of the time when I was growing up in my little village. There were a few of my peers walking around, clothed only in children slips, displaying what is known in my native Twi language as *funuma purudu*. The term stands literally for a protruding navel. Some of the navel hernias had indeed attained considerable sizes. Innocent as we were as regards the cause and also the potential life threatening complications of strangulation, we used to taunt them, indeed make fun of them.

Apart from the navel, the groin is another common hernia site. When a hernia first occurs the affected person may have a feeling that something has given way and may experience a little pain. The pain soon wears off. Later, a lump appears. This doesn't hurt and may get bigger on coughing.

The lump may from time to time disappear only to reappear again (as the herniating tissue slips back into place and then protrudes again.) In most cases hernias just cause discomfort and are a bit of a nuisance.

The real worry with hernias is that they may strangulate. Put another way, they could become stuck in the weak point in the muscles which in turn could lead to an interruption in its blood supply.

Without an emergency operation to release it and restore its blood supply, some of the tissue could die, leading to serious illness. As I was taught by the "medical experts" in my little village, it could lead to death.

RISK FACTORS

Following are some of the risk factors for the development of hernia.

- **Gender:** Men are particularly disposed to experience hernia of the groin because of their anatomy. (I shall not delve into further details.)
- **Inter-abdominal pressure:** Any activity that leads to a rise in the pressure within the abdomen such as lifting heavy objects, coughing, even straining on the toilet, can cause a weakness or tear in the abdominal wall, or force intestinal contents out through a weakness.
- **Previous surgery:** Surgery on the abdominal wall creates a vulnerable spot, which can later lead to a hernia. This type of hernia is also referred to as incisional hernia.

TREATMENT

Treatment usually involves surgery. Surgery may be through the traditional method of cutting and repair or by way of the so-called pin-hole surgery.

CHAPTER 13

High Blood Pressure

ONE DAY several relations of Rita, my wife, paid us a visit. In the course of the interaction one of our guests spotted the blood pressure measuring machine in the living room.

"Doc, can you please measure my blood pressure? I do not remember the last time I had it checked."

"No problem!" I replied. Without delay, I went into action to measure it. It read 115 over 70.

"Normal; no cause for concern!" I told him.

"Would you mind checking mine as well!" his other half requested.

"Of course not!" Like her husband, her pressure was also okay. Soon it turned out to be a kind of "children's game", for everyone present wanted to have his or her blood pressure checked!

Soon I would become not only a messenger of good news, but also of news not so pleasant—for, as it turned out, the blood pressure of one of our visitors was extremely high, requiring treatment as early as practicable!

Our visitor knew all along that his wife's blood pressure was high, a fact that had required her to take medication. What he was not aware of, however, was the fact that he had also developed the condition. (That is not to say that his wife had passed it on to him. No, high blood pressure is not, as it were, an infectious disease that our spouses or our neighbours can pass on to us. As we shall soon find out, we may inherit it from our parents, but that is as far as it goes.)

As it turned out, our relation had been living with high blood pressure, a veritable "time bomb", as it were, without being aware of it! That indeed is one of the disturbing aspects of high blood pressure.

If you and I visit a restaurant and eat food infested with the salmonella bacteria, our respective bodies would likely react in a matter of hours with nausea, vomiting and in some cases diarrhoea. Soon it would become clear to you and me that something is wrong with our body system. We would then take appropriate steps to reverse the situation. The situation, unfortunately, is different, when it comes to high blood pressure. One may indeed live with it for a considerable period of time without knowing it! Then, all of a sudden, one day, just like a time bomb waiting to explode, it does indeed burst out—sometimes in deep sleep. It could manifest itself as a stroke or a heart attack that could lead the individual never to awaken from sleep.

"He was fine, in real good spirits when he [or she] bade me goodnight!" the shattered spouse or relation might tell you.

Having said that by way of introduction, I shall give a brief overview of the condition.

Blood helps transport oxygen and nutrients to various parts of the body. On its journey back to the heart, it picks up the waste products of metabolism for further transport to the lungs, the liver, the kidney, etc.

The heart is an amazing muscular pump fixed in the chest to pump blood around the body. In order for the blood to be pumped around the body, pressure must be generated by the heart. Medical science uses the term *hypertension* when blood is forced through the arteries with an increased force.

Blood pressure is expressed as two numbers, for example "120 over 80". The top number is known as the systolic pressure. This stands for the pressure generated by the heart on beating. The bottom number, known as the diastolic pressure, stands for the pressure in the circulatory system when the heart is resting between beats.

A person's blood pressure is generally considered normal if it stays slightly above or below 120/80. A person whose systolic blood pressure is consistently 140 or higher or whose diastolic pressure is 90 or higher is generally considered to have high blood pressure.

CAUSES

In about 90% of cases, medical science has not found any reason to explain why someone's blood pressure is high. This condition is known as essential or primary hypertension. In the remaining 10 per cent of cases, there is an underlying cause. This is called secondary hypertension.

Some of the main causes for secondary hypertension are:
- chronic kidney diseases
- diseases in the arteries supplying the kidneys
- chronic alcohol abuse
- hormonal disturbances
- endocrine tumours

SYMPTOMS

As the example I cited at the beginning demonstrates, initially high blood pressure may not cause symptoms and go unnoticed until it leads to complications such as a stroke or heart attack.

In severe cases of the condition, some of the following symptoms could become apparent:
- headache
- sleepiness
- confusion
- coma

RISK FACTORS

Medical science has identified the following risks factors for the development of high blood pressure:

- Family Background: The condition tends to occur in families. For example, if your father or mother has the condition, you are also at risk of developing it as well.
- Obesity/Overweight: It has been established that people who are obese or overweight have a high risk of developing high blood pressure.
- Smoking: Apart from the more common risk factors associated with it such as lung cancer and other respiratory diseases, smoking has also been identified as a risk factor for the development of high blood pressure.
- Diabetes: Diabetes itself does not lead to high blood pressure. However, it has been established that the two conditions tend to occur together in the same individual.
- Kidney Disease: Certain types of kidney diseases lead the afflicted person to develop a high blood pressure.

TREATMENT

I have outlined above the possible risk factors for the development of high blood pressure. Avoiding the risk factors could help prevent disease.

If, despite such measures, the blood pressure remains high, treatment with medication would become necessary.

Such medication would need to be taken regularly and in some cases for the rest of the individual's life. Talking of taking medication on a regular basis! As a GP I have to keep on reminding my patients to do exactly that.

There are indeed some who, after the medication has led to a normalisation of the blood pressure, decide to stop taking it. This could eventually lead to a re-bound effect in which the pressure shoots up again.

MEDICATION

There are several medications in use. They are usually placed in groups.
Examples of the groups of medication in use are as follows:
- ACE Inhibitors
- Angiotensin-II receptor antagonists
- Beta-Blockers
- Alpha-Blockers
- Calcium-Channel Blockers Diuretics

I shall not consider the groups in detail. You may consult your family doctor for further details.

* * *

LOW BLOOD PRESSURE

Before I leave the area relating to our blood pressure, I shall impart some information on low blood pressure. In considering the possible complications of high blood pressure vis-a-vis low blood pressure, I usually tell patients with low blood pressure to be, as it were, happy that they have a low rather than a high blood pressure.

In the case of low blood pressure, the heart is pumping blood at a pressure below the average expected of a normal human being. Such individuals may feel dizzy and have the feeling that they might "pass out" especially on standing up. The reason behind this feeling may not be hard to figure out. The brain is very sensitive to oxygen and nutrients supplied by blood. When one stands up, the heart is required, at least momentarily, to pump blood with extra force in response to the altered position of the body. For the person with a low blood pressure the pressure generated by the heart may not be adequate.

CHAPTER 14

Heart Attack

T HE HUMAN HEART is indeed a masterpiece of creation.
It begins its pumping activity early in an individual's development and works dutifully around the clock. It works during the
day, as we go about life's activities, and at night when we are deep
asleep; it works in our joys and in our sorrows; it works in toil and
in ease; it works in the cold of the winter and the heat of summer.
Indeed, no matter the time of day, the season of the year, or the state
of our minds, this automatic pump fixed into our chests keeps dutifully pumping day in and day out to sustain us.

Assuming an average pumping rate of seventy per minute, our
heart pumps 100,800 times a day, or 36,792,000 times a year. In a
life spanning seventy years, that amounts to approximately 2.3 bil-
lion times.

Like all other organs of the body, the human heart is not free
from disease. This leads me to the term *heart attack* or *myocardial infarction*. The heart muscles do not derive their blood supply
directly from the blood being pumped from the heart's lumen or
inner cavity. Instead, the blood supply to the muscles of the heart
themselves is achieved by way of vessels known as the coronary
arteries and their tributaries or branches. These are located on the
outside walls of the heart.

As we might deduce from the above observations, the heart is a very busy muscular pump. As a result it needs a good supply of blood. Any interruption or blockage of the supply route of the coronary arteries may lead to the demise of the individual concerned.

A heart attack occurs when blood flow to part of the heart is blocked, often by a blood clot, causing damage to the affected muscle. If the blood supply is cut off for a short time, the muscles may regain vitality. On the other hand if the blood supply is interrupted for a considerable period of time, it could lead to irreversible damage to the heart muscles.

That in its turn could lead to the failure or the inability of the muscles to continue pumping blood. Depending on the extent of muscle damage, the situation could cause the heart to cease its pumping activity altogether, a situation which if not reversed within a short period of time, will lead to the death of the individual.

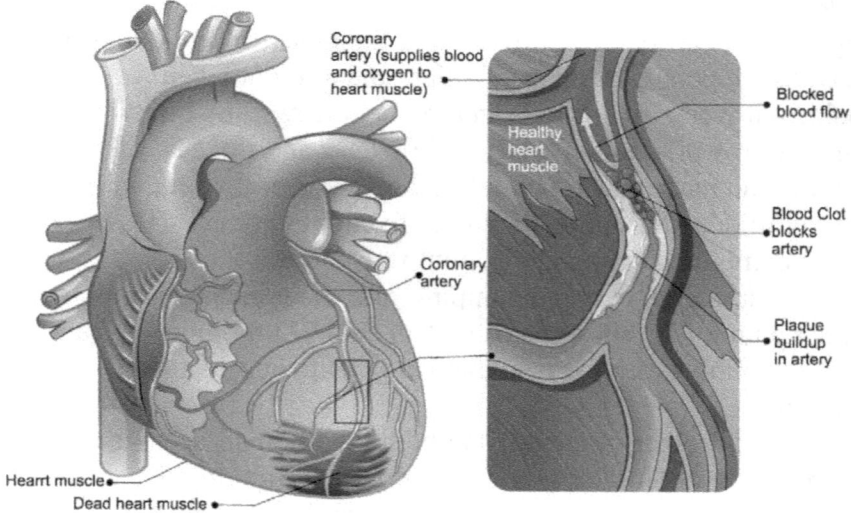

Coronary artery (supplies blood and oxygen to heart muscle)

Healthy heart muscle

Coronary artery

Blocked blood flow

Blood Clot blocks artery

Plaque buildup in artery

Hearrt muscle

Dead heart muscle

Heart Attack

RISK FACTORS

- **Smoking.** Smoking damages the interior walls of arteries including those supplying the heart. This favours the deposition of cholesterol and other substances on the walls of the vessels to form what is known as arteriosclerotic plagues. In time this could lead to a blockage of the vessel concerned.
- **High blood pressure.** Over time, high blood pressure can damage arteries, including those that supply the heart.
- **High blood cholesterol.** A high level of LDL ("bad") cholesterol, can favour the formation of arteriosclerotic plagues and in so doing lead to myocardial infarction or heart attack.
- **Family history of heart attack.** If your parents, grandparents or siblings have had heart attacks, you may be at risk, too. Your family may have a genetic condition that raises the risk of a heart attack.
- **Lack of physical activity.** Individuals who undertake regular exercise have a better cardiovascular fitness, which decreases their overall risk of heart attack. On the other hand, inactivity increases the risk of suffering a heart attack.
- **Obesity.** Being overweight raises the risk of heart disease because it is associated with high blood cholesterol levels, high blood pressure and diabetes.
- **Stress.** Studies have shown that those living a stressful lifestyle have an increased risk for developing a heart attack.

SYMPTOMS

Some symptoms associated with a heart attack are:
- Chest pain, usually a central, crushing pain, which may travel into the left arm or up into the neck or jaw, and persists for more than a few minutes. Unlike angina, the pain doesn't ease at rest. Sometimes the symptoms could be mild, which could be mistaken for indigestion.
- Shortness of breath or difficulty breathing.
- Sweating.

- Light-headedness.
- Dizziness.
- Palpitation.
- Nausea and vomiting.

TREATMENT

Heart attacks must be recognised and treated as quickly as possible because once a coronary artery is blocked, the heart muscle will die within four to six hours.

Signs to look out for in cardiac arrest

Before I leave the topic, I want to provide a brief overview of the measures that should be taken when we witness someone experiencing a cardiac arrest.

We should bear in mind that time is in the true sense of the word of the essence in such a situation. Each minute of delay reduces the chances of survival considerably.

Following are the signs to look out for in cardiac arrest:
- no palpable pulse.
- unconsciousness.
- apnoea (absence of breathing).

Emergency Measures in Cardiac Arrest

If available, call the emergency service. Whilst you wait you should undertake the emergency measure outlined below.

Immediate measures for resuscitation in cardiac arrest:

1 Hold the patient and shake him or her from the shoulders.
2. Ask him loudly in the ear whether he can listen to you.

3. Open the airway by lifting the chin upwards; this will facilitate easy breathing of the patient.
4. Check whether the patient is breathing. Look for chest movements and feel the air from the mouth of the patient. If effective breathing is present, then lay the person in a straight line with tilted chin.
5. If breathing is slow and not spontaneous, begin artificial (mouth-to-mouth) respiration immediately. It is important to check pulse and heartbeat at short intervals.
6. If there are signs of circulation, continue the mouth-to-mouth breathing for a while until spontaneous breathing is established. In the meantime it is important to keep on checking circulation at short intervals.
7. If no circulation is present, then compress the chest at the rate of about 100 per minute. Care should be taken to make a proper effort at compression. This should be forceful enough but not violent as rib injury may take place in such an instance. The current recommended chest compression to rescue breaths is 30:2. In other words 30 rapid chest compressions should be followed by 2 rescue breaths. This is the case for adults.
8. In case of **infants and children**, the ratio is 15:2 cycles when **two** rescuers are involved. If it involves one rescuer the ratio is as in adults, that is, 30:2.

CHAPTER 15

Stroke

⌒

THE BRAIN is the most complex organ in the body. It is divided into two sides, or hemispheres, each controlling the opposite side of the body and different areas of activity. The left hemisphere controls cognition (thinking) and language, plus movement and sensation on the right-hand side of the body. The right hemisphere controls functions involved in more visual-spatial skills, such as the ability to judge distances, size, form and where things are in space (which may affect skills such as map reading, for example), as well as movement and sensation on the left side of the body.

The brain regulates absolutely everything in the body—breathing, moving, sweating, sleeping, waking, feeling, thoughts, speech, etc. A constant supply of blood to deliver oxygen and nutrients to the brain cells is an essential pre-condition for the optimal function of the brain.

An interruption in the blood supply to the brain is termed a stroke. There are two types of stroke: ischaemic and haemorrhagic strokes.

- **Ischaemic stroke**. This is the more common of the two, accounting for around 80 per cent of all cases of stroke. This is the result of a blockage of one or more of the arteries supplying the brain with oxygenated blood, the blockage being caused by a blood clot.

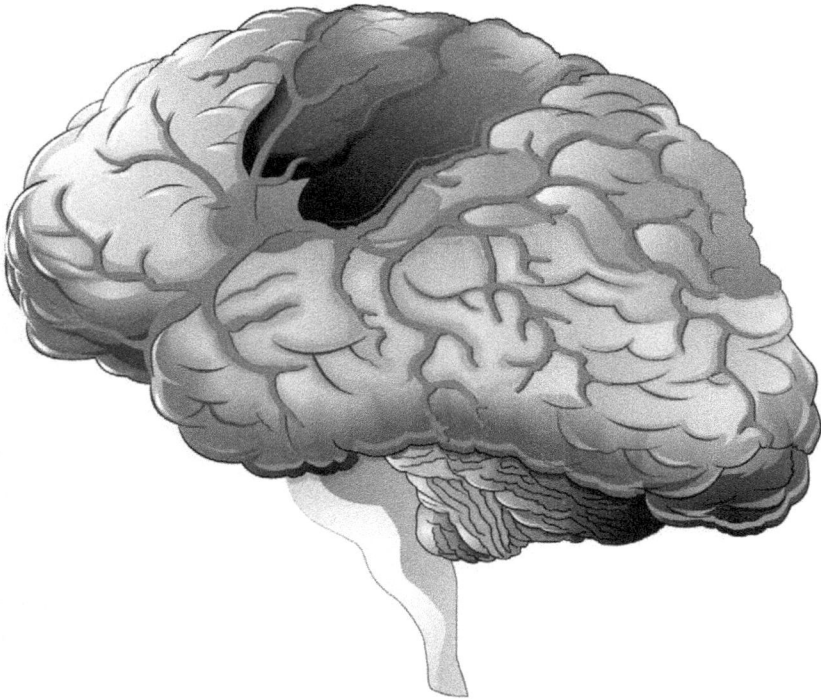

Bleeding into the brain in hemorrhagic stroke

- **Haemorrhagic stroke.** This occurs when one or more of the vessels supplying the brain ruptures or bursts out, causing bleeding in the brain.

Still on the subject of strokes—I want us to look at what is referred to as **transient ischaemic attack (TIA)** or mini-stroke. This involves a short-lived (usually less than 24 hours) disruption of blood supply to a part of the brain. Since the disruption is short-lived, so also is the disruption in the function of the affected part of the brain. This could be weakness of the limb, speech disruption, blurred vision etc. TIA does not lead to permanent brain damage. TIAs are important warning signs that could announce the occurrence of a full-blown stroke.

RISK FACTORS

Strokes and heart attacks share several common risk factors. These include:

- high blood pressure
- smoking
- obesity and
- inactivity.

SYMPTOMS

The symptoms of a stroke differ depending on the type of stroke and the part of the brain affected. The left half of the brain controls most of the activities of the right half of the body and the other way round. Thus a stroke affecting the left side of the brain could lead to loss of function on the right half of the body. The extent of loss of function depends on the extent of brain damage caused.

Symptoms usually set in suddenly, within seconds or minutes. Stroke and TIA symptoms may include:

- numbness, weakness or inability to move the face, arm or leg on one side of the body
- severe headache
- difficulty speaking
- sudden loss of sight in one eye or blurred vision
- confusion or difficulty understanding
- loss of balance or coordination
- seizures
- loss of consciousness

TREATMENT

Once brain cells have been damaged, they are irreparable. What can be done for a person who has suffered a stroke is to take measures to prevent another stroke or further strokes occurring in the future. Steps are therefore taken to treat the underlying cause of the stroke, for example high blood pressure.

In the acute phase of stroke, that is within the first 24-hours, treatment in a hospital, if available, is essential. I shall not go into the details of therapy here.

After the acute phase of therapy, the next stage is rehabilitation. It usually begins in the acute hospital, after about 48 hours of the occurrence. The aim of rehabilitation is to help the patient relearn skills lost following the brain damage brought about by the stroke. These skills can include coordinating leg movements in order to walk or carrying out the steps involved in any complex activity. Rehabilitation also teaches survivors new ways of performing tasks to compensate for any disabilities brought about by the stroke.

CHAPTER 16

Asthma

A STHMA is a disease that affects the respiratory tract. In asthma, the airways of the affected person suddenly begins to narrow. The narrowing of the airways in turn leads to laboured breathing and wheezing. One can imagine a situation when someone attacks us, and with both hands attempts to suffocate us.

The number of individuals suffering from asthma has increased significantly over the last several years. Experts associate the new development with increased atmospheric pollution as well as changes in diet and lifestyle over the years.

ASTHMA RISK FACTORS AND TRIGGERS

- **Family History**: Asthma tends to occur in families. It is thought that about three-fifths of all asthma cases are hereditary. Thus if your mother or father has asthma, you are predisposed to having the condition.
- **Sex**: Childhood asthma occurs more frequently in boys than in girls. Around age 20, the ratio of asthma between men and women is the same. By age 40, more females than males have adult asthma.

- **Cigarette Smoke**: Actively smoking or inhaling the smoke exhaled from a smoker (passive smoking) can trigger asthma. (Passive smoking has even been identified as a risk factor for new cases of asthma in preschool-aged children who have not already exhibited asthma symptoms.)
- **Obesity**: Though the reason is unclear, evidence suggests that obesity may contribute to or even cause asthma. This is because the prevalence of asthma is increased in the obese or overweight individuals.
- **Exposure to Pollutants and Chemicals**: Exposure to environmental pollutants such as exhaust fumes as well as chemicals used in farming, hairdressing and manufacturing, etc., can serve as risk factors for the development of asthma as well as triggers of the condition in the affected individual.
- **Allergy.** Exposure to one or more of the substances listed below could trigger asthma in the individual allergic to them:
  1. House dust mites
  2. Mould spores
  3. Pollen
  4. Pets
  5. Food or food preservatives
- **Infection**: Viral or bacterial infection of the respiratory tract could serve as a trigger to an asthma attack.
- **Exercise:** Earlier in the book I mentioned the benefits of exercise to the body. For some individuals, exercise, especially vigorous exercise (in particular in cold air) could serve as a trigger for an asthma attack.

SYMPTOMS

- Shortness of breath that leads the affected person to gasp for air.
- Tightness of the chest, a situation that leads the affected person to feel as if there is a band tightening around the chest.
- Wheezing, which is a whistling sound heard on breathing, resulting from airflow obstruction secondary to the narrowing of the airwaves.
- Coughing, particularly at night and early morning.

TREATMENT

The goal of treatment is to restore the constricted airways back to its original form. Basically there are two types of drugs in use.

Those of the first group act on the muscles of the constricted airways and cause them to relax, making it easier to breathe. These are also known as bronchodilators. The best known medication in this group is salbutamol.

The second group is made up of substances that act to reduce inflammation in the airways. This makes the airway less likely to react when exposed to asthma triggers. This group is made up mainly of steroids, for example beclomethasone.

Various combinations of the two types of substances are also available on the market.

In acute cases of asthma, the doctor may also dispense an injection with the goal of achieving swift relaxation of the respiratory muscles.

Where applicable, the doctor may also prescribe a short course of steroid tablets in an attempt to bring about a cure.

CHAPTER 17

Arthritis

⟨⟨⟨⟩⟩⟩

ARTHRITIS is an inflammation of a joint. This can occur suddenly in a previously healthy joint. In this case medical science speaks of acute arthritis. The condition may also persist after the initial manifestation. If this happens, the condition becomes chronic.

Chronic arthritis may cause the patient to experience episodes of worsening symptoms or flare-ups.

What is a joint?

Joints are points of connection between two bones or elements of a skeleton. With a few exceptions, joints are designed to allow movement between the bones and to absorb shock from movements like walking or repetitive motion. For the joints to move properly, they are endowed with a hard but slippery coating on their ends, known as cartilage. Healthy cartilage allows bones to glide over one another. It also absorbs energy from the shock of physical movement.

A tough membrane sac, the joint capsule, enclose the bones and other joint parts. Within the joint capsule is a thin membrane known as synovium. The synovium produces synovial fluid which serves the function of lubricating the joint to facilitate movement. In arthritis, the perfect order of the joint architecture is disturbed.

RIGHT KNEE   LEFT KNEE

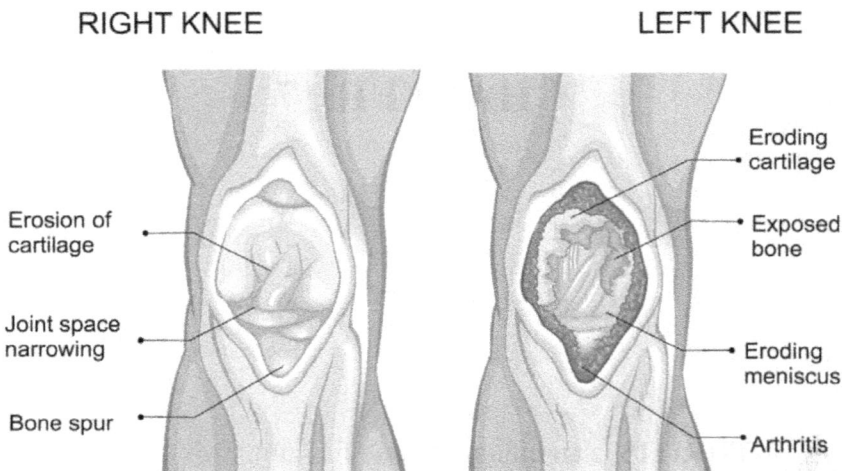

Knee-joint changes in arthritis

There are two types of arthritis: osteoarthritis and rheumatoid arthritis.

OSTEOARTHRITIS

Also known as wear and tear arthritis, osteoarthritis is a disease which becomes more likely as persons get older. In this condition the smooth cartilage that covers the end of bones begins to show signs of wear and tear. In the end, the fluid-filled space becomes smaller, causing the joint to be insufficiently lubricated. The wearing away of the joint cartilage may eventually expose the bone, leaving the surface of the now unprotected bone to rub directly against the opposing bone. This can lead to pain, in some cases severe or excruciating pain.

I try to explain osteoarthritis to my patients by comparing the human body to a brand new vehicle. Whoever has had the opportunity to drive a brand new automobile will have experienced the comfort of driving such a vehicle. In the first few months of its "life", it usually performs perfectly. In time, however, the brakes, the wipers, the clutch, etc., begin to show signs of wear and tear.

In the same vein, the human being, in his or her younger years, is usually fit and active. With the passing of time, however, his or her body begins to display signs of wear and tear, including the wear and tear of the joint surfaces.

Osteoarthritis most often occurs in the hands (at the ends of the fingers and thumbs), the spine (neck and lower back), and the knees, and hips.

RISK FACTORS IN OSTEOARTHRTIS

- **Age**: As was mentioned above, age is the main risk factor in the development of the condition.
- **Sex**: The condition is more common in women than in men.
- **Weight**: Being overweight increases the risk of osteoarthritis, in particular, osteoarthritis of the knee.
- **Previous injury:** an injury, surgery, earlier disease or repeated strain at a joint may lead to osteoarthritis later in life.

SYMPTOMS

Symptoms of osteoarthritis differ from individual to individual. Some people find the symptoms disabling whereas others may have few symptoms.

Symptoms may include the following:
- **Stiffness** in a joint especially on getting out of bed or sitting for a long time.
- **Swelling** and inflammation in one or more joints.
- **Constant or recurring pain** in a joint.
- **Crunching feeling** or the sound of bone rubbing on bone.

DIAGNOSIS

Your doctor may use the following steps to confirm the condition:
- History taking
- Clinical examination
- Blood investigation
- X-ray
- MRI-scan.

TREATMENT

- **Medication**: There is no medication to treat the underlying disease process. Instead, the goal of medical treatment for osteoarthritis (OA) is to reduce pain and stiffness and make it easier to remain active. Analgesics (painkillers) and nonsteroidal anti-inflammatory drugs (NSAIDs) are the most commonly prescribed osteoarthritis medicines.
- **Exercise**: Exercise, in particular, swimming, walking, and cycling, is known to have a favourable effect on alleviating the disease.
- **Weight control**: Weight reduction is important in the treatment of osteoarthritis. Weight loss can reduce the stress on weight-bearing joints, and in so doing limit injury and increase mobility.
- **Surgery**: In some patients surgery can help relieve pain and disability.
- **Use of prostheses**: In cases where joint degeneration has reached an advanced stage, surgeons may replace affected joints with artificial joints called prostheses. In general surgeons try to postpone the need for joint replacement as much as possible. Such joints usually last between 10 to 15 years; thereafter they need to be replaced.

RHEUMATOID ARTHRITIS (RA)

This is the second most common form of arthritis.

CAUSE

Earlier in the book, I explained the immune system, which defends us against infection and other diseases.

For reasons that cannot be explained the immune system sometimes turns against the same body it is there to defend. We may think of it as "friendly fire" as used in military jargon to describe the situation when an army fires accidentally on one of its own.

In the case of rheumatoid arthritis, the immune system attacks the tissues of the joints. This leads to inflammation of the joint. The inflammation causes swelling and redness in joints, and may make people feel sick, tired, and uncommonly feverish.

Persons suffering from rheumatic arthritis are subject to chronic joint pain with such acute recurrence that it can make their lives miserable. The joints eventually also become stiff, hampering smooth movement.

The most commonly affected joints are those at the ends of the fingers (closest to the nail), thumbs, neck, lower back, knees, and hips.

Compared with osteoarthritis, rheumatoid arthritis begins at a younger age than the former. It must be mentioned that apart from joints, rheumatoid arthritis can affect other parts of the body including the heart, lungs and digestive system.

RA can also occur in children. In this case, it is known as juvenile rheumatoid arthritis.

RISK FACTORS

- **Sex.** Women are more likely to develop rheumatoid arthritis than men.
- **Age.** As I just mentioned, rheumatoid arthritis can occur also in children. It is however most commonly observed in individuals between the ages of 30 and 60.
- **Family history.** As with many other medical conditions, one is at an increased risk of developing RA if other family members suffer from the condition.

- **Smoking.** Smoking has been identified as a risk factor for the development of RA.
- **Weight**: People who are obese or overweight are also at an increased risk of developing RA.

SYMPTOMS

- **Morning Stiffness:** A distinctive characteristic of rheumatoid arthritis is morning stiffness that lasts for at least an hour. In contrast the stiffness in osteoarthritis loosens up in about half an hour.
- **Swelling and Pain:** The joints swell up, turn warm and become tender. Indeed, swelling and pain in the joints must occur for at least 6 weeks before a diagnosis of rheumatoid arthritis is considered. The joint symptoms occur symmetrically in pattern, for example both knees, both wrists, the corresponding fingers of both hands, but may be more severe on one side of the body (unlike osteoarthritis where only one joint may be affected).
- **Specific Joints Affected:** RA almost always develops in the wrists and knuckles (the knee and joints of the ball of the foot are often affected as well). Concerning the fingers, RA affects joints at the base of the fingers while sparing joints at the fingertips (osteoarthritis on its part affects the fingertips).
- **Nodules:** In some cases of RA, inflammation of small blood vessels can lead to the development of pea-size nodules, or lumps, under the skin, especially near the elbow area.
- **Fluid Build-up in joints:** RA may lead to the build-up of fluid in the joints, in particularly in the ankles.
- **Flu-like Symptoms:** In the early stages of the disease cold or flu-like symptoms, such as generalised bodily aches and pains, fatigue and fever may be felt by the affected person.
- **Anaemia:** The condition may lead to shortage of blood in the affected person.

Symptoms in Children

In children, juvenile rheumatoid arthritis is usually preceded by high fever and shaking chills along with pain and swelling in many joints. A pink skin rash may also be present.

TREATMENT

There is currently no cure for the condition. The aim of therapy in RA is to reduce inflammation in the joints, relieve pain, prevent or slow joint damage, reduce disability and provide support to help the affected person live as active a life as possible. This is achieved through the following:

MEDICATION

There are several groups of medication in use:
- Painkillers, eg Paracetamol.
- **Non-steroidal anti-inflammatory drugs (NSAIDs),** e.g. Diclofenac.
- **Corticosteroids** (Steroids are usually only used on a short-term basis, as long-term use can have serious side effects).
- **Disease-modifying anti-rheumatic drugs (DMARDs),** e.g. Methotrexate.
- **Biological Treatment**: Biological treatments are newer forms of treatment for rheumatoid arthritis. An example is the group of medication represented by the tumour necrosis factor-alpha (TNF-alpha) inhibitors such as infliximab.

NON-DRUG TREATMENT

Following are some of the popular non-drug therapies for arthritic pain relief. They may be used alone, or in combination.

- **Hot and cold treatments.** Usually applied directly to the pain site; heat may be more useful for chronic pain, and cold packs provide relief from acute pain.
- **Exercise.** Keeping your joints and muscles moving helps in general fitness and can lead to decrease in pain.
- **Massage.** Massage can lead to relaxation of muscles and provide some arthritic pain relief.
- **Electrical stimulation.** Also known as transcutaneous electrical nerve stimulation (TENS), the therapy is delivered through a small device that sends a painless electrical current to large nerve fibres, generating heat that relieves stiffness and pain. The current also stimulates the release of endorphins, the body's natural painkillers.

LIFESTYLE CHANGES

The following lifestyle changes may favourably influence the course of the disease:
- A good and healthy diet.
- Losing weight in case of obesity.
- Smoking cessation.

SURGERY

Surgical treatment is employed in rheumatoid arthritis to relieve severe pain and improve the function of severely deformed joints that do not respond to medication and physical therapy. In some cases surgery may involve total joint replacement (arthroplasty).

CHAPTER 18

Diabetes

ONE DAY a middle-aged woman consulted me in my practice and began:

"Doc, I think there is something wrong with me."

"What then?"

"I have been feeling increasingly thirsty. Indeed, I am forced to drink almost all the time. That is not the end of the matter—I must frequently pass urine as well. It appears as if I have to drink water only to pass it out as urine!"

At this point in her narration the alarm bells, as it were, began to ring in my head. I was almost certain what was wrong with her; I wouldn't tell her immediately, however.

"There is certainly something wrong with you," I said. "We shall have to find out. You seem to have lost some weight as well."

"That is certainly the case. I have lost a few kilograms over the last several days. No wonder, for I have lost my appetite. I also feel tired all the time. Please Doc, help me, for matters certainly cannot continue like this!"

By now I knew exactly what her symptoms pointed to, namely, diabetes—what in several languages including my native Twi language is referred to as "sugar disease".

Knowing the type of person she was, I did not want to reveal my suspicions to her without first substantiating them with the relevant tests.

"We will have to conduct a few tests to find out what is wrong with you—first, you will need to provide us with a urine sample; next, we shall examine your blood."

"That's fine, Doc; I hope we are able to get to the bottom of the matter soon."

"We will do our best," I assured her.

As I expected, the tests confirmed my suspicion. Indeed, her symptoms were very typical of the onset of diabetes.

What, then, is Diabetes?

To go about our activities, we need energy, which is obtained from the food we eat. Through the process of digestion, the foodstuffs we eat are broken down into three basic components: glucose, amino acid, and fatty acid. These are eventually absorbed into our bloodstream.

We might consider glucose as a kind of fuel—petrol, diesel, or kerosene—that needs to be burned to power our body systems. For glucose to be effective, it must move into the cells to power the various reactions going on there.

The pancreas, a small organ located behind the stomach, is needed in the process.

Weighing approximately eighty grams, it serves two main functions. In the first place, it produces enzymes that help in the digestion of foodstuffs once they pass from the stomach into the small intestine. Most importantly, however, it produces two substances—insulin and glucagon, that help to regulate the level of glucose in the blood.

Without doubt, insulin, which helps to transport glucose from the bloodstream to the cells, is the more important of the two. After we have eaten to our fill and digestion and absorption has led to an elevation of the level of glucose in our bloodstream, the pancreas receives an order from the brain to release insulin into our bloodstream. The insulin thus released picks up the glucose circulating in the bloodstream for onward transport to the cells, like the letter carrier picking up our letters from the post office and depositing them in our letterboxes.

By means of one stone, insulin, the pancreas seeks to kill two birds. Firstly, it reduces the concentration of sugar levels in the blood and by so doing averts the harm that such high concentrations could have on the body in the end. Secondly, insulin ensures that the glucose reaches the parts of the body that need it, mainly, inside the cells.

In diabetes, or "sugar disease", the pancreas may either completely cease to produce insulin or may not produce insulin in a sufficient quantity. It may well be the case that the body cells of the affected person cannot react properly to insulin produced by the pancreas.

In a person suffering from **Type1 Diabetes** the cells in the pancreas responsible for insulin production are destroyed. It is thought by medical science that the destruction of the pancreas cells is due to an autoimmune disease (remember what I said earlier when I explained the immune system). It is thought that a virus infection or an environmental factor serves as a trigger to spark the autoimmune reaction.

In the case of **Type 2 Diabetes**, either the pancreas cannot produce enough insulin or the body cells of the affected person cannot react properly to insulin.

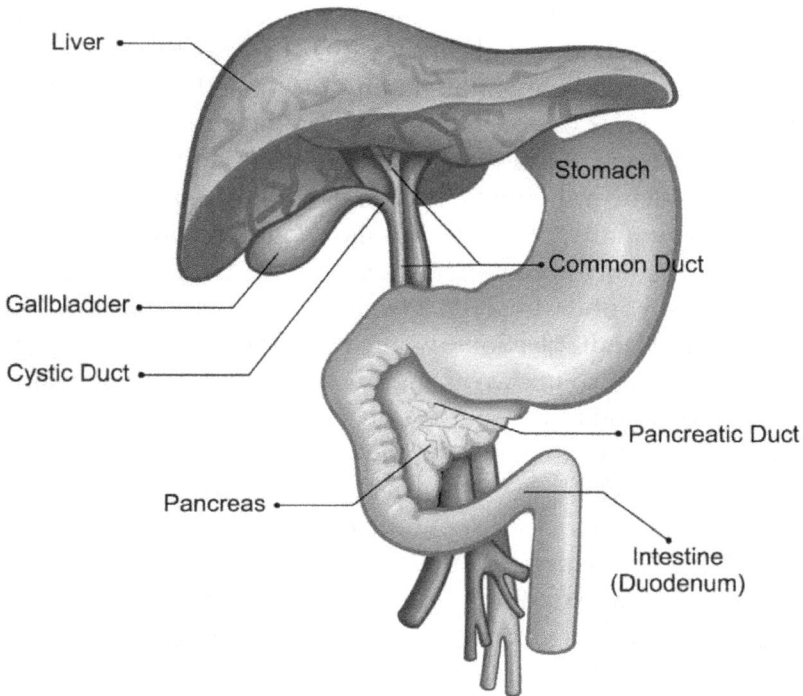

Liver •
Stomach
Common Duct
Gallbladder •
Cystic Duct •
Pancreatic Duct
Pancreas •
Intestine
(Duodenum)

Position of the pancreas in the body

RISK FACTORS FOR TYPE 2 DIABETES

- **Obesity**: Obesity or being overweight is a major risk factor for the development of Diabetes Type 2. Previously, the condition was generally associated with adults. As the number of overweight children increases in many societies, so also, unfortunately, does the number of children who increasingly are being diagnosed with the condition.
- **Lack of exercise**: With the advent of automobiles, the remote control, the computer, computer games, etc., we have increasingly become inactive. Inactivity coupled with the availability of abundant food in our refrigerators may lead us to overfeeding which in turn could lead to overweight which in turn could lead to the development of Type 2 Diabetes.
- **Unhealthy eating habits**: Earlier I touched on the concept of a balanced diet. Bad or unhealthy eating habits—eating too much fat, too much carbohydrate (starchy food), and not enough fibre increases the risk of developing Type 2 diabetes.
- **Family history:** As in the case of high blood pressure, diabetes seems to occur in families. It does not follow automatically that because your father or mother has the condition you are also going to get it. You only need to remember that you are more susceptible to getting it in order to adopt a healthier lifestyle.
- **Gestational Diabetes:** Some women develop diabetes during pregnancy. This is also known as *gestational diabetes*. In the majority of cases, the condition returns to normal after birth. Studies have shown that these women stand the risk of developing Type 2 diabetes later in life. Such women are thus advised to avoid exposing themselves to the risks just outlined.
- **High Blood Pressure**: As I mentioned in the chapter on high blood pressure, the two conditions seem to go together. If you have been diagnosed with high blood pressure, your risk of developing Type 2 diabetes is higher than that of the general population.

SYMPTOMS

As we saw earlier, my patient presented us with some of the typical symptoms of the disease. These include:
- Feeling thirsty all the time.
- Having to pass urine all the time.
- Weight loss.
- Feeling tired and exhausted.
- Loss of appetite.

TREATMENT

Type 1:

As we learnt above, in the person with Type 1 diabetes, the body cannot produce insulin at all. Treatment is by way of insulin. Insulin, when taken in tablet form, is destroyed by acids in the stomach. Consequently, the main route of application is by means of injection. Attempts are being made to produce insulin that can be inhaled so as to spare victims the need to inject insulin.

Type 2 Diabetes:

As we saw earlier, in patients with Type 2 diabetes, the pancreas is either not producing sufficient insulin to meet the demands of the body, or the body cells cannot react properly to insulin (medical science speaks in this case also of insulin-resistance).

Treatment in this case is by means of tablets that help to activate the remaining pancreatic cells to increase insulin production. Some of these patients may have to inject insulin in addition to taking the tablets.

We learnt about the risk factors in developing the disease. In some instances blood sugar levels can be restored to normal levels without even the need for medication. Instead, the patient takes steps to reduce the risk factors that lead to the condition—reducing weight, following the proper diet and undertaking regular exercise.

LONG TERM EFFECT OF DIABETES

Diabetes that isn't well controlled can lead to long-term problems for the patient. The elevated blood glucose associated with the condition can lead to the damage of blood vessels which in turn can lead to: heart and kidney disease, stroke, impotence and nerve damage.

CHAPTER 19

Epilepsy

$\sim$

AT THE TIME I was growing up in my little village, one of our fellow residents suffered from epilepsy. The great majority of the population were either completely illiterate or at best semi-educated. Hardly anyone of us had any idea as to the underlying cause of the disease. Consequently we fell victim to the then prevailing belief that the disease could be passed on to anyone who happened to come too close to the afflicted person at the time he or she was experiencing a fit. Thus, whenever the victim of the disease suffered a fit, whoever happened to be near him, made for the hills instead of going to his aid.

CAUSES

Our brains are made up of billions of nerve cells. The nerve cells transmit impulses from one to the other. They do so by way of chemicals known as neurotransmitters. There are two types of neurotransmitters; one type leads to an increase in impulse transmission, whereas the other inhibits the process. In normal life the activities of the two transmitters are co-ordinated in such a manner as to lead to stability in brain activity. A disturbance in the delicate balance could lead to epileptic fits.

RISK FACTORS

Below are some of the factors that can bring about a disturbance in the delicate balance in neurotransmitter activity in the brain alluded to above.

- **Genetic abnormality:** Medical science has observed that some types of epilepsy tend to run in families. This has led to the suspicion of genetic abnormality as one possible cause of the disease.
- **Head injury:** Head injuries sustained in accidents may lead to seizures or epileptic fits. This is particularly so when the injuries involved happen to be severe.
- **Prenatal injuries:** When we are developing in our mother's womb, our brain cells are very susceptible to adverse changes in the womb environment brought about either by maternal illness or behaviour. For example, some types of infection contracted by an expectant mother, or habits such as smoking, alcohol consumption as well as the abuse of certain drugs, if continued through the pregnancy, can adversely affect the unborn child and lead eventually to epilepsy in later years.
- **Environmental factors:** Exposure to lead, carbon monoxide, and certain chemicals, should it persist for a considerable period, could lead to the development of epilepsy.
- **Alcohol:** Long-standing alcohol abuse can increase a person's risk of developing epilepsy.
- **Disease:** Epilepsy can be a secondary manifestation of a primary condition such as brain tumour, meningitis, HIV, etc.
- **Other factors:** sleep deprivation and stress could lead to epileptic fits in an individual.

TREATMENT

Medication: There are several groups of medication in use for the treatment of epilepsy. Treatment depends on several factors including the age of the affected person, how often the seizures occur, how severe they are as well as the overall health of the affected person.

Readers are advised to contact their own doctors in regard to the treatment options available.

Surgery: In some instances surgery, the details of which I shall spare the reader, is employed in the treatment of epilepsy.

CHAPTER 20

Sexually Transmitted Diseases

GENERAL OVERVIEW

- Sexually transmitted diseases (STDs) are infections that can be transferred from one person to another through sexual contact.
- STDs are sometimes referred to as sexually transmitted infections (STIs).
- They are most often caused by viruses and bacteria, though they may also be caused by other organisms such as fungi, pubic lice, scabies etc.
- STDs affect men and women of all ages and backgrounds, including children.
- STDs have become more common in recent years, partly because people are becoming sexually active at a younger age, are having multiple partners, and do not use preventive methods to lessen their chance of acquiring an STD.
- STDs can be present in an individuals but cause no symptoms (eg Chlamydia, gonorrhoea, genital herpes). The affected can then pass the disease on to their sexual partners.
- Many STDs can be passed from a mother to her baby before, during, or immediately after birth.
- A person may obtain more than one type of infection at a time.

For example, one may be infected at a single sexual contact with both gonorrhoea and chlamydia.

I will now consider in some detail some of the common STDs around.

CHLAMYDIA

Chlamydia is caused by the bacterium, Chlamydia trachomatis. The disease can affect women and men as well as children during their passage through the birth canal. Symptoms usually appear approximately 7 to 21 days after infection and differ for men, women and children. In men Chlamydia can cause inflammation of the urethra (the passage through which urine passes to the outside of the body). This in turn can result in a stinging feeling when passing water. The disease can also lead to a discharge from the male genital organ and possible itchiness as well as pain. Finally it could also lead to pain in the testicles.

As in men, the disease can also lead to a stinging feeling in women when passing water as well as being accompanied by unusual genital discharge. The disease can lead the affected female to experience pain during intercourse as well as experience bleeding between periods. Infection in an expectant mother could lead to premature birth.

Infants can contract the disease during birth. An infection could lead to the following symptoms: conjunctivitis (inflammation of the eye), breathing problems, chest infection (pneumonia).

DIAGNOSIS

Diagnosis is done by performing a swab test of the infected area and examining it in the laboratory for evidence of infection.

TREATMENT

This is by means of suitable antibiotics, e.g. Doxycycline and Zithromax. It is recommended that the spouse of the affected person is also treated.

GONORRHOEA

The condition is caused by bacteria called Neisseria gonorrhoea. It can affect both sexes. In women, the cervix or the neck of the womb is the most common site of infection. The disease can also spread to the uterus (womb) and fallopian tubes. This can lead to the blockage of the fallopian tubes which in turn can lead to infertility!

In women the early symptoms of gonorrhoea are often mild, and many women who are infected have no visible symptoms of the disease. In the female symptoms include: a painful, burning sensation when urinating, a yellowish or bloody discharge from the genital organ, intermenstrual bleeding and abdominal pain.

Symptoms in the male are clearer than in the female. They include a burning sensation when passing urine and a yellowish-white discharge from the male genital organ.

Gonorrhoea can be passed from an affected expectant mother to her new-born infant during delivery.

DIAGNOSIS

Diagnosis is made through detection of bacteria in samples taken from the urethra or cervix.

TREATMENT

The condition is treated with antibiotics such as penicillin, cefixime and ciprofloxacin. Treatment should be extended to the spouse of the affected person. As with Chlamydia, further testing is recommended once treatment has ended to check whether the infection has cleared.

HERPES GENITALIS

This is caused by the herpes simplex virus (HSV). It is a highly contagious condition. It is transmitted primarily through physical and sexual contact. During birth, an infected mother can pass the condition on to the new-born during his/her passage through the birth canal. This could lead among others to the development of herpetic meningitis.

SYMPTOMS

The outbreak may be accompanied by other symptoms such as:
- Swelling and tenderness of the lymph nodes in the groin area.
- In women, vaginal discharge and painful urination.
- In men, a possibility of painful urination if the lesion is near the opening of the urethra.
- Fever.

TREATMENT

There is no cure for the herpes simplex virus; once infected, patients will remain a carrier for the rest of their lives. Timely treatment (within five days of symptoms starting) with antiviral medication will reduce the severity and duration of symptoms. A five-day course of treatment is usual, but may be extended by a few days if blisters are still forming. Examples of this group of medication are aciclovir, famciclovir and valaciclovir.

HIV/AIDS

HIV has become a household name. HIV invades and destroys the immune system, which as I have mentioned in several places in this book, is a defence system in place in our body to, among other things, protect the body from infection. The result of this is that the affected person becomes prone to many different types of diseases.

We might well imagine what would happen to a country should it be invaded by outside forces, just at the very point in time when its entire military force is incapacitated by disease.

RISK FACTORS

The virus is found in bodily fluids such as blood, sperm and vaginal secretions, and can pass through little scratches that may be present or occur during sexual intercourse. Consequently intravenous drug users and people with many different partners are particularly at risk of contracting the disease.

SYMPTOMS

Although they vary considerably, the symptoms include:
- fever
- diarrhoea
- night sweats
- weight loss
- swollen glands
- the feeling of being generally unwell.

DIAGNOSIS

The diagnosis is made when the HIV antibody is found in the blood. The test is not usually positive until 6 to 12 weeks after infection.

TREATMENT

That HIV has until now no effective cure is a well-known fact, and may be superfluous to mention here. Therapy currently is aimed at the improvement of the quality of life and its prolongation. Several medications aimed at achieving this are currently on the market. It is beyond the scope of this book to look at the various types of medication in detail.

GENITAL WARTS

Also known as condylomata acuminate, it is a very contagious condition caused by the human papilloma virus (HPV). As we shall see later when we come to treat cancer, some strains of this virus can lead to changes in the cervix which in turn can lead to the development of cervical cancer. Up to nine months can pass from the time of infection to the actual development of warts. About a third of cases of genital warts may resolve without treatment after six months. Rarely, they can develop into cauliflower-like growths.

SYMPTOMS

These include the following:
- Red, pink or grey-coloured cauliflower-shaped lesions in the genital and anal area that look raised or flat. The abnormal growths may develop into large clusters and expand into huge masses very rapidly.
- Tiny papules on the shaft of the penis.
- Discomfort and itching in the affected areas.
- Mild cases of warts are usually painless. In severe cases, they may cause severe pain.

DIAGNOSIS

A diagnosis is made when a characteristic lesion is visible. By swabbing the skin with 5 per cent acetic acid, 'invisible' warts will emerge as white-coloured patches.

TREATMENT

Treatment of genital warts depends on their size and location.
- Chemicals such as imiquimod and podophyllotoxin may be used to remove visible warts.
- Cryotherapy : This involves the freezing of genital warts, using liquid nitrogen.
- Where available, laser therapy can be used.
- Surgery can be used to remove genital warts, in particular those that have assumed large sizes.

SYPHILIS

The disease is caused by bacteria called Treponema pallidum. The route of transmission of syphilis is almost always through sexual contact though it can also be transmitted from mother to child in the womb or during birth. It can be potentially life-threatening because after infection, the bacteria is transported through the bloodstream to various parts of the body. In the end it could adversely affect vital organs such as the heart, brain, nervous system and spine.

DIAGNOSIS

This is made through the detection of the micro-organism or the detection of antibodies in the blood.

SYMPTOMS AND STAGES OF DISEASE

There are three stages of the disease:
- Stage 1: This occurs up to the first twelve weeks of the infection. During this period one or more red lesions could be observed in the genital area. The lesions usually disappear after a week.
- Stage 2: Symptoms could be observed up to about six months after the time of infection. These may include the following: a red rash on the chest, back, arms, legs, hands and soles of the feet; high fever; muscular fatigue as well as a general feeling of discomfort.
- Stage 3: If the disease is not identified and treated, it will disappear for a while only to return later, sometimes up to twenty years later. At this more advanced stage of the disease, the symptoms could include heart failure, paralysis, insanity which in turn could lead to the death of the patient. (If we sit down to consider the fact that a disease contracted several years ago through sexual contact could cause us serious problems twenty years later we would indeed make every effort to ensure that our bodies do not become infected due to careless behaviour.)

TREATMENT

Syphilis: is treated with penicillin, administered by injection. Other antibiotics can be used for patients allergic to penicillin. Left untreated, it could damage the heart, the brain, eyes and bones. In some cases these effects could lead to death.

PART 4

WOMEN'S HEALTH

CHAPTER 21

Menstrual Disorders

IN THIS CHAPTER I will deal with menstrual problems and problems related to menopause. Before I do that, I want briefly to explain the menstrual cycle. In our present discussion, we will assume the cycle has an average duration of twenty-eight days, although it may deviate a few days from individual to individual.

The cycle in effect is the female body's way of preparing itself to accommodate the would-be product of the union referred to earlier. The expected union not having materialised, the womb decides, albeit with a heavy heart, to discard the material put in place to receive the newcomer.

Depending on the individual involved, the menstrual bleeding may last anywhere between three and seven days (or more). When the bleeding is over, the brain sends instructions to a structure located at its base, the pituitary gland, to begin releasing into the bloodstream a hormone it had all along been producing and storing in its body. This hormone on its part carries the name follicle-stimulating hormone, or FSH. FSH in turn instructs one of the two ovaries of the womb to order one of the several follicles it is harbouring to grow into maturity. The follicles are tiny liquid-filled sacs, each containing an egg. At birth, each girl already has several follicles. They remain dormant until she reaches maturity.

Usually during each menstrual cycle, only one follicle grows into maturity. In rare instances, however, two or more may do so simultaneously and release their eggs into the womb.

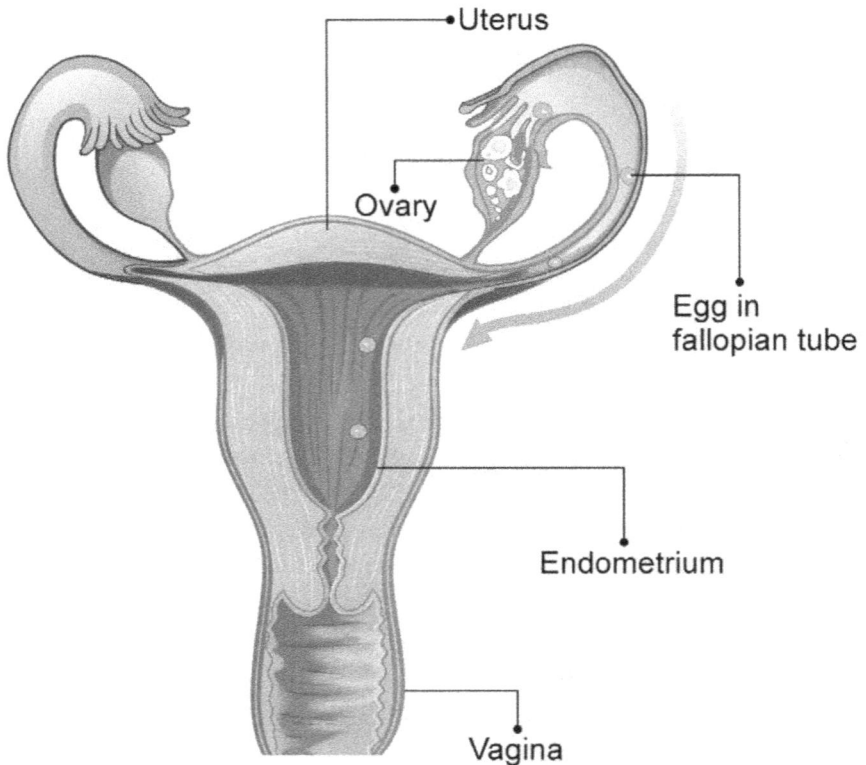

Mechanism of ovulation in the menstrual cycle

There are two ovaries on each side of the womb. For the sake of fairness, the follicles release at alternating months from each ovary. Prior to the release of the matured egg into the womb, the maturing follicle releases a considerable amount of a hormone known as oestrogen into the bloodstream. Under the influence of oestrogen, the lining of the womb grows increasingly thicker.

Just about the middle of the 28-day cycle, that is, round about the fourteenth day, the matured egg drops into the womb. We call this event ovulation.

The important role the follicle plays does not end with ovulation. Now re-named corpus luteum, it begins to release, in addition to oestrogen, another hormone, progesterone, into the bloodstream. Together, both hormones support and maintain the thickened walls of the uterus in anticipation of the possible implantation of the fertilised egg within it.

In the absence of fertilisation, the corpus luteum degenerates in about fourteen days. With decreasing levels of oestrogen and progesterone in the bloodstream brought about by the degeneration of the corpus luteum, a new menstrual cycle soon sets in.

Having explained the mechanism of menstruation, I will now turn to some of the common problems and disturbances that could affect the menstrual cycle.

AMENORRHEA

The age of onset of menstruation in a girl varies from individual to individual, depending on several factors. Some girls start menstruation as early as 8 years whereas others have to wait until they are around 16 years of age.

It is generally agreed that by the age of 16 every girl would have experienced her first menstruation. If this does not happen, the resulting condition is referred to by medical science as primary amenorrhea.

There are instances when a girl /woman who has all along not had any problem with her period, all of a sudden stops to menstruate. If this condition persists for six consecutive months, the doctors refer to the condition as secondary amenorrhoea. (One has to keep in mind that it may well be due to a pregnancy, of course.)

DYSMENORRHEA

A certain degree of pain or discomfort accompanies even the normal menstrual cycle. Medical science speaks of dysmenorrhea or menstrual pain when the discomfort and pain is bad enough to interfere with the normal daily life of the individual concerned.

The pain typically occurs in the lower abdomen and/or pelvis and can radiate to the back and along the thighs, lasting somewhere between 8 and 72 hours. It may be a constant dull ache or occur as cramps before or during menstruation or both. Headaches, diarrhoea, nausea and vomiting may accompany it.

Severe menstrual pain can be a sign of an underlying disease such as endometriosis and fibroids.

In endometrioses, the cells that line the cavity of the womb and that are shed during each menstrual cycle, are also found in places outside of the womb. During each menstrual period, the tissue outside of the womb, like that inside the womb, responds to the hormones that regulate the menstrual cycle. This leads to a breakdown and bleeding of the tissue in the same way as those lining the walls of the womb. This can lead to inflammation and pain.

MENORRHAGIA

This refers to prolonged or excessive menstrual bleeding that occurs at regular intervals. In most cases no cause can be found. However, there may be an underlying cause such as endometriosis, fibroids or even womb cancer.

INTERMENSTRUAL BLEEDING OR SPOTTING

This refers to bleeding of variable amounts that occur between regular menstrual periods. These may have several causes including hormonal imbalance, infection, fibroids, etc.

POLYMENORRHEA

In this case bleeding occurs in regular intervals of less than 21 days.

OLIGOMENORRHOEA

This is irregular or infrequent periods. Menstruation can occur anywhere between every six weeks and six months.

PREMENSTRUAL SYNDROM (PMS)

Premenstrual Syndrom, PMS for short, is a condition that occurs about ten to fourteen days before the onset of menstruation. It involves physical and emotional symptoms that may include bloating, pressure on the pelvis, headaches or migraines, difficulty concentrating, irritability, mood swings and increased craving for food.

The degree to which PMS occurs is different from woman to woman—some women may experience none, some, or many PMS symptoms. Also for each individual woman, the symptoms may be worse in some months than others.

For those women who experience mood swings, this may well be a time of emotional instability—an emotional state in which the woman can easily become angry with those who come into contact with her.

CHAPTER 22

Fibroids

A **LSO KNOWN** as myomas, fibroids are benign (not cancerous) tumours found in the muscular wall of the womb or uterus. They are quite common occurring in about a third of all women. Many of the affected women live with it without knowing it, for indeed in many cases fibroids are not accompanied by any symptoms. That, unfortunately, is not the case for all women, for fibroids do cause problems for many.

CAUSES

Medical science has not been able to explain exactly why some women develop fibroids and others do not. There is general consensus among the experts however as to the role of the hormone oestrogen.

Oestrogen plays an important role in the function of the female body. The level of oestrogen falls after the menopause. It has been observed that the size of fibroids in women decreases after the menopause. This has led to the conclusion that oestrogen, even if it does not cause it, at least facilitates the growth of fibroids.

Fibroids vary in their location, shape and size. Also, whereas some women develop a single fibroid which may assume large sizes, others develop many small fibroids.

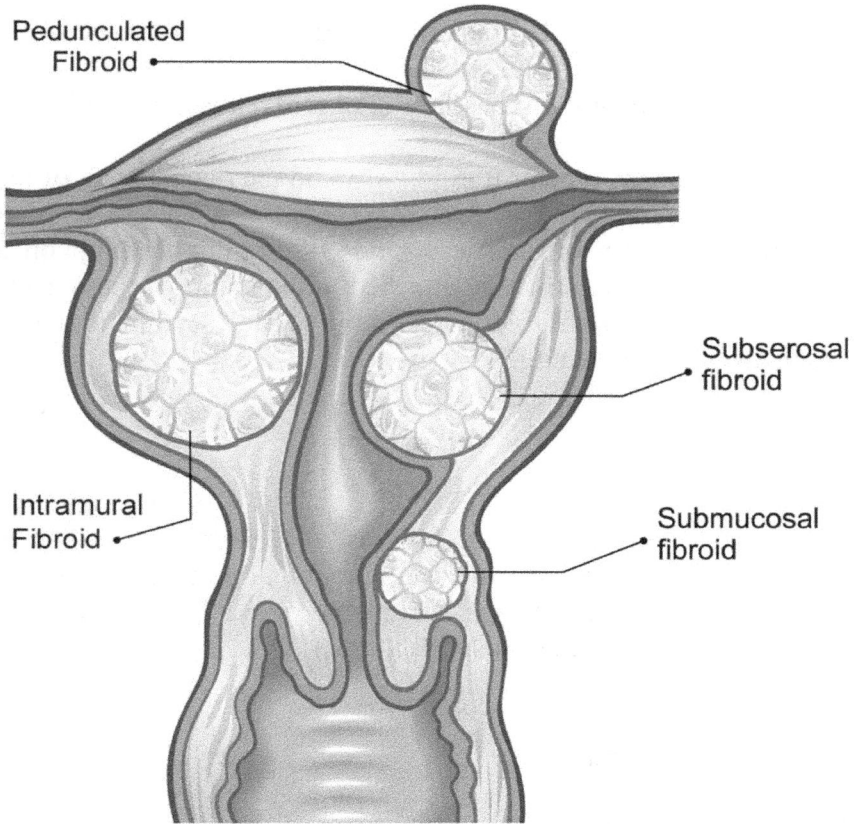

Types of Fibroids

TYPES

Based on their location relative to the womb, fibroids are divided into four main types:

- **Submucous fibroids**. These grow in the hollow space within the womb. By virtue of their location these types of fibroid can adversely affect a pregnancy. This is especially the case should the pregnancy implant on it. In such a situation the fetus is in danger of not receiving an adequate blood supply which in turn could lead to a miscarriage. Ultimately, submucous fibroids could result in infertility of the affected woman.

- **Intramural fibroids**: Theses are fibroids located within the muscle of the uterine wall.
- **Extramual**: This type of fibroid grows on the outside wall of the womb.
- **Pedunculated fibroids:** These kinds of fibroids develop on a 'stalk' or stem-like structure attached to the inside or the outside of the uterus. These fibroids can become twisted, leading to severe pain and heavy bleeding.

SYMPTOMS

What are the signs that point to fibroids? As I mentioned earlier, in several women they produce no symptoms at all. Usually they begin to cause problems when they assume large sizes. (That is not to say that small fibroids do not cause problems.)

Menstrual Disturbances

They can be in the form of:
- Increased menstrual bleeding which in turn can lead to anaemia.
- Prolonged menstrual bleeding.
- Increased menstrual frequency.
- Inter-menstrual bleeding (bleeding between the normal menstrual period).

Abdominal Pain

Fibroids, particularly large ones, may lead to bloating and/ or abdominal discomfort.

Low Back Pain

Fibroids that have assumed large sizes can lead to lower back pain.

Urinary Problems

The womb lies not far from the urinary bladder. Fibroids, in particular large fibroids, may result in the compression of the urinary bladder which in turn can lead the woman to urinate frequently.

Constipation

Fibroids can also press against the rectum (the end of the large intestine) and lead to constipation.

Other related problems

Huge fibroids may create the impression of the affected person being pregnant. In some societies it could lead to all sorts of rumours among neighbours, particularly if it is not treated early. One can imagine the psychological impact that it could have on the affected woman.

Problems with childbirth

As I mentioned above, fibroids, especially those found within the womb, can cause problems in the pregnancy, especially so when the pregnancy implants on it. This can lead to inadequate blood supply to the fetus which in turn can lead to miscarriage. In the end this type of fibroid can lead to infertility. Even if it does not lead to infertility, they can lead to complications during the pregnancy. These can be in the form of threatened miscarriage, miscarriage, premature delivery, etc.

Fibroids, if they are located in the birth canal, can make normal delivery impossible.

DIAGNOSIS

This is mainly by means of a clinical examination (pelvic examination) followed by an ultrasound scan (if available).

TREATMENT

Most fibroids do not require treatment. Treatment is usually needed if the fibroids are causing some of the symptoms listed above, pain or bleeding, or if the fibroids are large or rapidly growing.

Medication

Some types of medication act on the fibroids with the aim of reducing their size and preventing them from growing any further. Other types of medication are used to treat the bleeding associated with the condition.

Surgery

Surgery is considered where medication does not lead to the expected results. The choice of surgery depends on the type and size of the fibroid and include:
- Myomectomy: This involves the removal of the fibroid and the preservation of the womb. This path is usually pursued where the fibroids involved are small and also where the woman desires to have children. (The fibroids may return at a later date, however.)
- Hysterectomy: This involves the complete removal of the uterus.

CHAPTER 23

Female Infertility

I F A COUPLE should fail to conceive during a year of unpro-tected intercourse, medical science refers to the couple as being infertile. Infertility can be caused by a problem with the man or the woman, or both.

Female reproductive problems account for 40 per cent of all cases of infertility, while 40 per cent are assigned to the male. In the remaining 20 per cent, medical science is at a loss as to the cause.

Yet, in several societies, the female is usually the first person assigned blame when couples find it difficult to conceive.

In my native Ghana, the pressure on the female can, in such a situation, be enormous. We have a family set up that can be regarded as a community. Children are not looked upon as belonging to the couple involved but to the community, the extended family as a whole. When a marriage after a while fails to produce children, the extended family members of both individuals have a tendency, sooner rather than later, to point accusing fingers at the woman.

In this chapter I will consider some of the factors that may lead to female infertility. Male infertility will be treated in the following chapter.

CAUSES OF FEMALE INFERTILITY

OVULATION PROBLEMS

It takes two to tango! The sperm of the male may be active, agile and willing to tango with the egg of the female, but if the eggs are absent in the womb at the time Mr Sperm gets there no tango can take place. Eggs are released by the female in the process of ovulation. What factors can lead to problems of ovulation?

One of the culprits identified is the so-called Polycystic Ovary Syndrome (PCOS). This condition affects about 5% to 10% of women of reproductive age. Some of the features present in a female displaying signs of the syndrome are obesity (overweight), female masculinisation (when women display features that make them appear to look like men), acne, irregular periods, inability to ovulate. How far the above symptoms develop in an individual is different from woman to woman.

TUBAL PROBLEMS

After ovulation, Princess Egg needs to travel through the fallopian tube to meet Prince Sperm to join together in marriage. In some instances, several factors working either alone or together prevent that from happening.

Following are some of the factors that may cause problems to the egg in its journey through the fallopian tube:
- Endometrioses
- Pelvic adhesions
- Pelvic Inflammatory Disease
- Blocked Fallopian tube

UTERINE PROBLEMS

After Mr Sperm and Miss Egg have sealed their marriage bond, they need a home to settle in and develop their relations. The uterus comes into play here. Several conditions in the uterus can prevent this from happening; if in their attempt to settle in the womb their peace is disturbed by unruly elements, the new residents may decide, prematurely, to vacate their new residence (leading to miscarriage).

One of the conditions in the uterus that could lead to such a situation is the presence of fibroids. Fibroids, in particular those within the womb, as we noted earlier, can lead among other things to the improper implantation of the fetus on the wall of the womb and lead to miscarriage, not only of one pregnancy but several others.

AGE-RELATED FACTORS

With age, it usually becomes increasingly difficult for a woman to conceive.

DIAGNOSIS

A doctor suspecting female infertility would do the following to confirm his/her suspicion (I shall leave out the details):
- History, including menstrual and pregnancy history
- Clinical examination
- Blood investigation
- Ovulation tests
- Laparoscopy (to determine endometrioses and adhesion)

TREATMENT

The following are some of the treatment options:
- **Induction of Ovulation**. If the inability to ovulate is the cause of infertility, the doctor will prescribe medication with the goal of overcoming the problem.
- **Intrauterine Insemination**: This is a fertility procedure whereby sperm are washed, concentrated and injected directly into a woman's uterus. In natural intercourse, only a portion of the sperm are able to travel up the woman's genital tract to the fallopian tube to bring about fertilisation. Intrauterine insemination increases the number of sperm in the fallopian tube; that in turn increases the chance of fertilisation taking place.
- **IVF**: This is a term which in the meantime has become generally known. You may speak to your doctor about the details.

CHAPTER 24

Pregnancy-related issues

~

NORMAL COURSE OF A PREGNANCY

Someone has said that at the time of our birth we are already nine months old. This is indeed true, for from the moment of conception, the complex genetic blueprint for every detail of human development—sex, hair and eye colour, height, and skin tone—are already mapped out.

By approximately the fifth week of the union, the individual's heart has begun to beat. By the end of the fourth week, the spinal cord, muscles, and nerves have become apparent; so also the arms, legs, eyes, and ears. During the last six months of pregnancy organ systems continue to refine themselves.

At the end of nine months the incredible events are complete and a child is about to be born. The normal position for the baby as it prepares for birth is head down and facing the mother's back.

SIGNS AND SYMPTOMS OF A NORMAL PREGNANCY

Having spoken of the normal course of pregnancy by way of introduction, I shall now move on to outline some of the common signs and symptoms of a normal pregnancy. It should be noted that symptoms may vary from woman to woman; also, some of the symptoms are similar to the discomforts that a woman may experience prior to a normal menstruation.

Missed Period: This is the most obvious early pregnancy symptom. This could be caused by other medical conditions, but if it is followed soon by some of the symptoms outlined below, it is likely due to a pregnancy.

Breast Tenderness: A tender, swollen and a slightly sore breast. Some women may also notice their nipples darken in colour.

Nausea and Vomiting: Nausea and vomiting, especially in the morning, may be experienced very early in the pregnancy, as early as a week into the pregnancy.

Fatigue, Dizziness and Fainting: For some women one of the early signs of pregnancy is the feeling of being tired for the most part of the day. While this may force them to go to bed early, they may also find it difficult to wake up in the morning. In addition to feeling tired all the time, some women may also often feel dizzy and feel like passing out.

Frequent Urination: Pregnancy results in an increase in body fluids that has to be processed by the kidneys. The expansion of the uterus, on its part, exerts constant pressure on the urinary bladder. Both factors together lead to frequent urination of the pregnant woman.

Heartburn: Many women experience heartburn (also known as indigestion or acid reflux) during the pregnancy. This is a burning sensation that usually extends from the bottom of the breastbone to the lower throat. The greatly expanded uterus or womb exerts pressure on the stomach which in turn leads to the reflux of acid present in the stomach into the oesophagus or gullet to cause the burning sensation just alluded to.

Constipation: Constipation is a common problem during pregnancy. During pregnancy, the body produces more female hormones than usual. One of the hormones, progesterone, leads to a relaxation of the bowel muscles making them less able to move food and bodily waste along, causing constipation. In the last months of pregnancy, the growing baby also exerts pressure on the bowels, which in turn leads to constipation.

Lower Back Pain: This is due among other factors to the increase in weight that goes with the pregnancy and the change of posture that comes about as a result of the pregnancy.

PREGNANCY COMPLICATIONS

Having outlined some of the signs and symptoms of a normal pregnancy, I shall now turn my attention to consider some of the complications, some of which can be serious, indeed, life-threatening, to both mother and child.

ECTOPIC PREGNANCY

The uterus is there to nourish a pregnancy. Unfortunately, in some instances, after fertilization has taken place, the zygote or the fertilized egg implants outside the lumen of the womb. This results in an ectopic pregnancy or a pregnancy that is "out of place". In about 95% of cases, ectopic pregnancies involve the fallopian tube. Apart from the fallopian tube, the fertilized egg may also implant in the ovary, cervix or in the abdomen. Such areas are incapable of providing the needed space and nourishment required for the normal development of the pregnancy. As the fetus grows and expands, eventually the organ containing it bursts. This can lead to severe bleeding and a life-threatening situation to the would-be mother.

Signs and Symptoms: Symptoms of an ectopic pregnancy can be difficult to diagnose because they are similar to those of a normal early pregnancy—a missed period, breast tenderness, nausea, vomiting, etc.

The first real warning signs of an ectopic pregnancy are often pain or vaginal bleeding. Most women describe the pain as sharp and stabbing. It can be felt in the pelvis, abdomen and in some cases even in the shoulder or neck. (Blood built up from the ruptured ectopic pregnancy could irritate nerves supplying those areas.)

Apart from pain and bleeding, the following could also point to an ectopic pregnancy:

- vaginal spotting
- dizziness or fainting (caused by blood loss)
- low blood pressure (also caused by blood loss)
- lower back pain

Risk Factors: In theory any woman can be affected. The risk however is highest for women who are 35 years old and above and have had:

- a previous ectopic pregnancy
- previous surgery on a fallopian tube
- pelvic inflammatory disease (PID)

Treatment: Treatment of an ectopic pregnancy varies, depending on how medically stable the woman is and the size and location of the pregnancy.

Doctors may treat an early ectopic pregnancy by:

1 Injection: Medication could be injected to stop the further growth of the embryo.
2. Surgery: This is particularly the case in an emergency situation involving life-threatening bleeding.

MISCARRIAGE

Miscarriage is the loss of the baby during the earlier weeks of pregnancy. The World Health Organisation (WHO) defines it as being up to 23 weeks of the pregnancy and 500 grams in weight.

There are variations in the period of time set by the WHO from country to country. This can vary from 20 weeks till up to 28 weeks of pregnancy. Early miscarriage is mainly due to the fetus failing to develop normally. Later miscarriage on its part is more likely to be the result of the placenta not functioning properly or a weak cervix. Symptoms include bleeding, but this is not always the case and about half of all women who bleed in the early stages of pregnancy do not go on to miscarry.

PRE-ECLAMPSIA

Pre-eclampsia is a condition related to increased blood pressure and protein in the mother's urine. It typically starts after the 20th week of pregnancy. The causes are not entirely clear, but are thought to be related to defects in the placenta (after-birth).

Risk Factors: Some mothers are more at risk of developing pre-eclampsia.

These include mothers with:
- a first pregnancy
- diabetes
- previously diagnosed hypertension
- multiple pregnancy (twins or triplets, etc.)
- a previous history of pre-eclampsia.
- a history of kidney disease.

Treatment: Regular blood pressure and urine checks will help detect preeclampsia. Once the condition is diagnosed, frequent monitoring of blood pressure, urinary protein excretion and weight become essential. If the condition worsens and the mother or baby or both is/ are at risk, labour may be induced or a caesarean section performed.

GESTATIONAL DIABETES

Gestation diabetes is a condition in which women who have not been known to have diabetes before, exhibit high blood glucose levels during pregnancy. As we saw earlier on, insulin is needed to transport sugar from the bloodstream to the cells. In pregnancy, there is a higher demand on the pancreas to produce insulin. In some women, the pancreas is not able to meet the increased demand for insulin.

Risk Factors: These include obesity, women aged over 35 years as well as women with a previous history of gestational diabetes

Treatment: Treatment for gestational diabetes will depend on the severity of the diabetes. The goals of treatment are to keep blood glucose levels within normal limits during the duration of the pregnancy, and to ensure the well-being of mother and the developing baby.

- **Diet:** Mild forms can be treated with diet, in particular by decreasing the intake of simple sugars and fats.
- **Exercise**: Regular physical activity is sometimes used to keep blood sugar levels lower because contracting muscles help stimulate glucose transport.
- **Insulin**: When the above measures fail to keep blood glucose levels within an acceptable range, insulin injections are resorted to.

Gestational diabetes usually disappears following delivery though women who experience the condition have an increased risk of developing Type 2 Diabetes later in life.

BLEEDING

Bleeding during pregnancy could be scary and should be taken seriously. Fortunately such bleeding doesn't always have a serious underlying cause.

Bleeding during pregnancy could however have serious underlying causes. These may include:
- ectopic pregnancy
- threatened miscarriage
- placenta previa and
- placental abruption.

Placenta Previa: In this condition the placenta is fixed at a lower than usual position in the womb, and lies over the opening of the cervix. Placenta previa will often correct itself during pregnancy. In case it fails to do so and it leads to bleeding, doctors will assess the severity of the condition and decide on either emergency caesarean section or on monitoring the patient in hospital for a while.

Placental Abruption: In this case, the placenta has come away from the wall of the womb. It occurs usually from about 28 weeks onwards and usually causes sudden severe abdominal pain with some dark red bleeding or clots. It may necessitate in some cases an emergency caesarean section. If the symptoms are less severe, a short period of monitoring in hospital may be all that is required.

CHAPTER 25

Menopause

O**NE DAY** one of my patients consulted me to report a peculiar condition that had been plaguing her for a while. The symptoms, she went on, included hot flushes that would suddenly descend on her. According to her, her body would in such moments feel very hot, as if in a hot oven. In such moments she would feel like pulling off her clothing, even if she happened to be walking on the street! The hot sensation, she continued, could suddenly go to the other extreme, and she would experience a sensation of coldness. She would feel like she was freezing—indeed, as if she were living in the middle of a severe winter! She also reported night sweats, sweats that were so extreme that her bedding became drenched in sweat! Partly as a result of the night sweats, she was forced to turn and turn in her sleep, something that was disturbing not only her sleep, but that of her husband as well.

"At times," she said, "my husband is so scared by my behaviour he thinks I may be going crazy!"

The symptoms displayed by my patient are among some of the typical ones associated with menopause.

What is Menopause?

In a previous chapter, I explained the menstrual cycle and its role in reproduction. Menopause in the strictest sense of the word is the permanent cessation of menstruation.

A woman is generally considered to have reached menopause when she hasn't menstruated for twelve months. The time of onset of menopause differs from woman to woman. For most women it occurs between the ages of 40 and 56 years.

There is usually a transitional period, the pre-menopausal period. Again, this can differ from woman to woman. In some women it can last several years; in other women it can be a matter of just a few weeks. The premenopausal period is characterised by irregular menstruation.

For the majority of women the onset of menopause or the transition to that stage is uneventful. As in the case of the abovementioned patient, menopause can present symptoms that in some cases can be scary and burdensome.

SYMPTOMS

My patient has already described three typical symptoms of the condition, namely hot flushes, night sweats, and sleep disturbance.

Other symptoms are:
- dry skin, including drying of the genital organ
- thinning of the skin
- itching
- joint pains
- mood changes which can lead to irritability, anxiety, nervousness and depression
- fatigue (feeling tired all the time)
- weight gain

MANAGEMENT OF MENOPAUSE—RELATED SYMPTOMS

Hormone Replacement Therapy (HRT): Hormone Replacement Therapy (HRT) is an option for providing relief from symptoms of menopause. Since many problems associated with the menopause are believed to be due to reduced oestrogen levels, the main component of hormone replacement therapy (HRT) is oestrogen, although some preparation may include progesterone.

Because it replaces female hormones produced by the ovaries, hormone replacement therapy minimizes menopause symptoms such as night sweats, hot flushes, mood swings, genital dryness, etc.

One of the disadvantages of HRT therapy is that it is associated with a slightly increased risk of developing blood clots, ovarian cancer and breast cancer in some susceptible women over the age of 50.

Natural Remedies: Some women choose to avoid HRT and prefer to resort to natural remedies in the form of vitamins, herbs, soy, and dietary changes to help with the symptoms of menopause.

• **Remifemin**, obtained from Black cohosh, which is part of the buttercup family of plants, is purported to relieve symptoms of menopause—depression, night sweats, hot flushes, anxiety and irritability.
• **Phytoestrogens** or plant estrogens are natural compounds similar to oestrogen that help to alleviate a variety of menopausal symptoms. Phytoestrogens are found in foods such as fruits, sprouts, red clover, yogurt, lentils and spinach.

PART 5

MEN'S HEALTH

CHAPTER 26

Benign Prostatic Hyperplasia (BPH)

T HE PROSTATE gland is a chestnut-shaped organ found only in the male. It is located beneath the bladder and surrounds the urethra, the tube through which urine passes from the bladder into the penis. It plays an important role in the male reproductive system, producing the liquid that provides not only nutrients for sperm, but also protects and helps to drive them forward in the process of ejaculation.

In the young adult, the prostate gland weighs around 20g. As one grows old, the prostate gland tends to increase in size. Eventually it could grow to weigh as much as 150g. Often the condition is benign or non-cancerous and is referred to as benign prostatic hypertrophy (BPH).

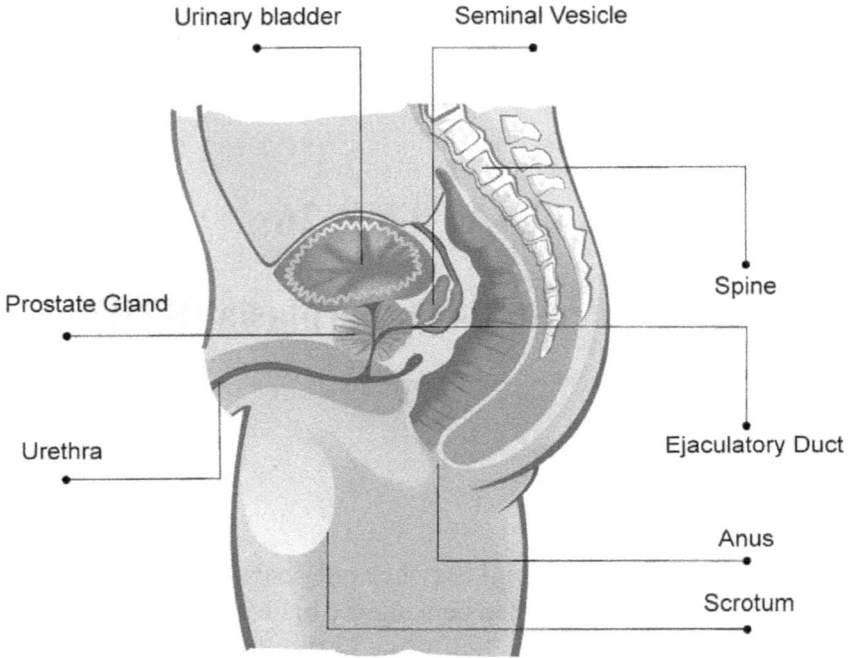

Position of the prostate gland in the body

SYMPTOMS

As the prostate grows, it constricts the urethra which in turn could lead to some of the symptoms listed below:

- Urinary frequency, i.e. the need to empty the bladder often, not only during the day but also at night, something which in turn could lead to sleep disturbance.
- Difficulty in starting the urine flow.
- Dribbling after urination.
- Decrease in the size and strength of the urine stream.

TREATMENT

- **Medication:** The medication in use either reduces the size of the enlarged prostate or relaxes the muscles in the prostate gland. Either way, the aim of therapy is an easing or elimination of the obstruction of urine through the urethra.
- **Surgery:** Surgery is resorted to where medication has not brought the desired effect. The standard surgical procedure is referred to as transurethral resection of the prostate gland (TURP). It involves the use of a device equipped with a small camera and a small sharp instrument which enables the surgeon to cut away excess prostate tissue.
- **Emergency Surgery in BPH**: BPH can sometimes lead to a medical emergency situation referred to as acute urinary retention. This is a situation whereby the enlarged prostate gland leads to a complete obstruction or blockage in the passage of urine to the outside. This usually necessitates surgical intervention whereby a cut is made on the lower abdominal wall and into the bladder. A catheter, suprapubic catheter, is then put in place to help drain the urine.

CHAPTER 27

Impotence /Erectile Dysfunction (ED)

C~

IN AN EARLIER chapter I mentioned that despite the general inclination of society to apportion blame to the woman when couples are infertile, medical science has established that the fault could equally lie in the man's court.

Before I move on further to consider the causes of male infertility I wish to clarify a point—impotence (erectile dysfunction) should not be confused with male infertility. Indeed, one can be potent, that is, be in a position to perform the role expected of him in a marriage relationship, and still be infertile.

MECHANISM OF ERECTION

An understanding of the mechanism at work in the male to ensure a proper erection is important to an understanding of erectile dysfunction, the situation when the mechanism, as it were, grinds either to a complete or partial stop.

The male sexual organ has two chambers. Both chambers are filled with a spongy tissue known as corpora cavernosa, within which are muscles, fibrous tissues, spaces, veins, and arteries. The spongy chambers are wrapped in a thick membrane called the tunica albuginea. The rod-like male sexual organ is endowed with a tube, the urethra, which serves as a passage for urine and sperm.

Sensory and mental stimulation trigger the erection process. Several body parts work together to ensure it works. In the first place, the brain sends a message of sexual arousal through the nervous system to the male sexual organ. This message causes the muscles of the corpora cavernosa to relax. At the same time, the size of the artery, the vessel carrying blood from the heart to supply the organ, expands to twice its original size. As a result, the volume of blood it carries increases to about sixteen times compared to what it was before.

Simultaneous to the tremendous increase in the blood supply to the male sexual organ, the veins, the vessels responsible for transporting blood away from the penis, is blocked; blood is thus trapped and cannot escape. This mechanism leads to a stiffening and enlargement of the male sexual organ.

The tunica albuginea, the thick wall wrapped around the corpora cavernosa, also plays an important role in helping to trap the blood and in so doing sustain the erection.

There is mechanism in place to ensure the process of erection reverses after a while. The process begins with the contraction of the muscles of the organ. This reduces the inflow of blood to the levels that persisted before the erection process. Simultaneously, the blockage on the walls of the veins lifts to allow outflow of blood.

CAUSES OF ERECTILE DYSFUNCTION (ED)

Several factors can come into play to cause the dysfunction of the mechanism outlined above. These include the following:

Hormonal conditions

Examples of hormonal conditions that can cause ED include:
• **Hypogonadism**—a condition that affects the production of the male sex hormone, testosterone, causing abnormally low levels.

- **Hyperthyroidism** (an overactive thyroid gland)—where too much thyroid hormone is produced.
- **hypothyroidism** (an underactive thyroid gland)—where not enough thyroid hormone is produced.
- **Cushing's syndrome**—a condition that affects the production of a hormone called cortisol.

Anatomical conditions

Examples of anatomical conditions that can cause ED include:
- **Peyronie's disease**—a condition that affects the tissue of the male sexual organ.
- **hypospadias** - a seldom anatomical abnormality that results in the urethra developing on the underside of the male sexual organ.
- **Diabetes**—by adversely affecting the blood vessels of the body, diabetes negatively influences the mechanism of erection.
- **Smoking**. The effect of smoking could be compared to that of diabetes—smoking adversely affects the vessels.
- **Alcohol Abuse**—it does so mainly by adversely affecting the nerves.
- **Spinal Cord and Brain injuries**. From the mechanism of erection outlined above, one can easily understand why a brain or spinal cord injury could have an unfavourable effect on the erection mechanism.
- **Diseases that affect the Nervous System**: stroke, multiple sclerosis.
- **Side effects of certain drugs**, notable some blood pressure medication and anti-depressants.
- **Effects of recreational drugs,** for example cocaine, ecstasy, marijuana.
- **Stress and mental disorder.** Indeed, a certain degree of vitality in the individual is required for the system to function. We all know how we feel after we have spent eight, ten, twelve or sometimes more hours on our feet engaged in a very strenuous activity. Stress in this case does not apply only to physical stress; indeed, emo-

tional stress, even problems in the relationship, could, if only in the short term, negatively influence the system.
- Ageing. Erectile dysfunction is most common in men older than 65. With increasing age comes increasing damage to the vessels of the body, including those that supply blood to the male genitalia. This in turn can lead to erectile dysfunction.

TREATMENT

ELIMATION OF UNDERLYING HEALTH CONDITIONS

If erectile dysfunction is caused by an underlying health condition, such as heart disease or diabetes, treating the condition may lead to an improvement or even complete resolution.

LIFESTYLE CHANGES

The symptoms of ED can often be improved by making lifestyle changes to reduce the impact of known risk factors for the condition. These may include the following :
- **Weight reduction in case of overweight**
- **giving up smoking**
- **cessation or moderation of alcohol consumption**
- **avoiding the use of recreational drugs**
- **regular exercise**
- **reducing stress**

HORMONE THERAPY

If deficiency of certain hormones is causing ED, substituting the affected hormone through synthetic alternatives may lead to an improvement.

RESORTING TO AN ALTERNATIVE MEDICATION

In some cases ED could be due to the side effects of medication. In that case one has to consult his doctor to discuss alternative medication. One is however advised not to stop taking prescribed medication on his own volition unless after consultation with his doctor.

DRUG THERAPY FOR ED:

The most commonly used medication are the so-called phosphodiesterase-5 (PDE-5) inhibitors. They work by temporally increasing the blood flow to the male sexual organ.

The three common ones in use are:
- **sildenafil** – Viagra.
- **tadalafil** – Ciali
- **vardenafil** – Levitra

As in the case of any typical medication, they are not free of side effects. One is therefore strongly advised to take them only if prescribed by a doctor.

CHAPTER 28

Male Infertility

$\backsim$

HAVING considered the causes of erectile dysfunction, I shall now tackle male infertility in the broader sense. Indeed ED is only one factor among several possible causes of the condition.

For the male to be fertile several conditions need to be met:
• In the first place, the individual involved must be in a position to produce mature sperm.
• Next, that individual should be in a position not only to have an erection, but also to sustain it so as to be able to discharge the sperm into the female.
• The sperm should be in sufficient quantity and have the quality to be able to bring about fertilization.

Failure to meet any of the above conditions could lead to infertility.

CAUSES

Erectile Dysfunction—this has already been discussed above.

Testicular factors: there are situations where the testes, which can be described as a factory for the production of sperm, produce low quantity and/or poor quality sperm. Following are some of the factors that can lead to such a situation:

- **Cryptorchidism**: During the time a male person is developing in his mother's womb, the testes first form in the stomach. In the course of time, they descend into the scrotum. Latest, by the time of birth, both testes should have done so. There are instances however when either one or both testes fail to do so. Within one year after birth, about 80% of the testes that had failed to descend do so retrospectively. Undescended testes are associated with reduced fertility. This is because sperm require a temperature lower than that found in the body to develop (the temperature in the scrotum is lower than that of the body).
- **Hydrocele**. I mentioned earlier the case of the resident in my little village carrying a huge hydrocele of the scrotum around the little settlement. A hydrocele testis can adversely affect the production of sperm.
- **Hormonal Problems**. Deficiency of the male hormone, testosterone, can lead to a decrease in sperm production which in turn can lead to reduced fertility.
- **Smoking** has been shown to reduce both sperm count and sperm motility.
- **Alcohol**. Excessive intake of alcohol can lead to a low sperm count and have a detrimental effect on male fertility.
- **Stress, emotional or physical,** can each or in combination cause low sperm count, which in turn can lead to reduced fertility.

TREATMENT

As in the case of erectile dysfunction, treating the underlying cause of male infertility may lead to a reversal of the situation. Should the condition persist, you should contact your doctor to discuss the best way forward.

PART 6

CANCER

CHAPTER 29

Definition, General Symptoms, Diagnosis & Treatment of Cancer

 ~

C ancer is indeed a common word which among other things conjures up fear and apprehension in many—and not without cause. Cancer is indeed one of the most common causes of death.

What then is cancer? I will attempt an explanation of the term *cancer* in a manner that, hopefully, everyone can understand.

Our bodies are made of cells. The cell indeed is the basic unit, or building block, of life. All living things are made up of one or more cells. Organisms may exist as single cells (unicellular), or, like ourselves, as a group of cells working together (multicellular).

The cells in our body are constantly undergoing wear, tear and death. For life to continue, cells must be able to divide or replicate to replace the dead ones. Usually the cells divide in a controlled manner. The parent cell, in a process known as mitosis, divides into two so called daughter cells. Each daughter cell after a while becomes a parent cell that in turn divides into two daughter cells; and so on, and on, the process continuing as long as life continues.

In cancer, this control mechanism has gone out of control. Put in a simple way, cancer cells, the moment they begin to divide, continue unabated to divide, divide and divide. What makes cancer cells a nuisance to the body is the fact that they are incapable of performing the functions of the original cell from which they developed.

Let us take white blood cells as an example. The white blood cells, as we saw earlier, are there to defend the body against outside invaders. White blood cells that have turned cancerous, known also as leukaemia cells, whilst swimming in abundance in the liquid part of the blood (plasma) are, to put it bluntly, good for nothing—just good for nothing!

Yet another feature of cancer cells—they can, without exaggeration, be described as insatiable gluttons! Always hungry for food, they voraciously consume a considerable portion of whatever nutrients their poor victims are able to supply to their bodies.

If only the cancer cells would restrict themselves to the organ in which they developed. Indeed, if only, for example, cancer cells that have developed in the pancreas would confine their destructive activities to that organ only.

It is said that the moment you offer some human beings one centimetre, they go on to demand one metre. The same thing can be said of the cancer cells. For example, cancer cells of the pancreas would sooner rather than later leave the walls of the pancreas and begin to infiltrate, penetrate and invade neighbouring tissues and organs.

One might assume that would be the end of the matter, but no! Ultimately, cancer cells of the pancreas could move to settle in the brain, the liver, and the bones! How did they get there, one might ask? Well, the answer is simple—through the bloodstream and the lymphatic system.

One might imagine that cancer cells, on arrival in their new hosts, would stay quiet and enjoy the kind hospitality accorded them. That unfortunately is seldom the case. On the contrary, no sooner have they settled into their new environment than they resume their malicious activity of uncontrolled division. Soon, instead of brain cells growing in the skull of the victim, pancreas cells will be doing so as well.

GENERAL SYMPTOMS OF CANCER

Different types of cancer produce different symptoms, depending on the organ involved. There are however symptoms that most cancers share in common. Here are a few of them:

- **Persistent Fatigue (feeling tired all the time).** Fatigue is not unique to cancer. Several other factors—stress, anaemia, malnutrition, lack of vitamins, chronic infectious diseases such as HIV etc.—could also lead to the condition. Still, one should have cancer in mind, especially in case fatigue persists over a considerable period of time.
- **Weight Loss.** If you happen to be overweight and have actively contributed to a reduction in weight, more grease to your elbow! If, on the other hand, you have all of a sudden, inadvertently, lost a substantial amount of weight, you are advised to have a health check to rule out cancer and other diseases associated with weight loss.
- **Loss of Appetite,** should it linger on for a while, could point to various kinds of diseases including cancer.
- **Pain.** Several conditions can cause pain to the body. In cancer, pain is usually not an early sign of the disease. Instead, it is generally associated with advanced stages of the disease, especially at the stage when it has gained in size or spread to other parts of the body, in particular the bone.
- **Fever.** Earlier in my discourse I dealt with fever and cited the various conditions that can lead to fever. Fever, usually, is a transitional condition. Should the condition however persist for long, it could be a sign of cancer, especially blood cancer (leukaemia) or cancer that has spread to other parts of the body.
- **Night sweats.** Unexplained sweating in the night could be due to several conditions—menopause, infections, diabetes, but also cancer (such as leukaemia).

GENERAL PRINCIPLES OF CANCER DIAGNOSIS

There are several general principles applied by medical science in cancer diagnosis. One of the most important tools is screening.

Screening: Cancer cells are normal body cells gone astray. The most effective way to contain them is to fight them at the very early stage of development, long before they are able to spread to neighbouring as well as distant organs.

Now, how can you and I, ordinary human beings with limited resources at our disposal, become aware that at any time of our existence, some of our cells, cells that until then have dutifully served us, have all of the sudden turned into cancer cells poised to destroy us? Screening is the only effective tool available to medical science that has the means of detecting the problem—in other words, that can detect and identify the presence of cancer cells in our body as early as possible. It enables the doctor to detect cancer cells in order to come to a decision to take the appropriate action to curtail or eradicate them. It is indeed true that as far as the treatment of cancer goes, time is of the greatest essence.

Screening aims to find, attack and destroy cancer cells as early as possible before they are able to destroy their victim.

GENERAL PRICIPLES OF CANCER TREATMENT

Before I consider a few selected cases of cancers in detail, I want to consider the general principles behind the treatment of cancer. As I mentioned earlier, cancer basically is uncontrolled cell division that leads to the development of tumours.

- **Surgery**: Removal of the tumour, especially in the early stages, will help prevent the spread to other organs. In an advanced stage, a stage when cancer has spread to other parts of the body, surgery may still be needed especially if the growth is pressing on neighbouring organs thereby preventing the organs involved from performing their functions. For example, if cancer is compressing

the gullet, preventing the victim from swallowing, surgery could be performed to alleviate the situation.
- **Radiation Therapy:** This involves the use of high-energy x-rays or other types of radiation to kill cancer cells or keep them from growing.
- **Chemotherapy**: In Chemotherapy, the patient is prescribed drugs with the goal of stopping the growth of cancer cells either by killing them or preventing them from dividing.

One form of the three types of therapy outlined here does not exclude the other. In other words, the said types of therapy can be combined in various ways with the goal of achieving the best possible results.

I will now move on to consider a few common cancers in some detail.

CHAPTER 30

Breast Cancer

 ❧

A LTHOUGH men can develop breast cancer, the disease is about a hundred times more common in women than in men.

RISK FACTORS

Medical science has identified several risk factors in the development of breast cancer. Some can be classified as low risks, others as high. I will only name a few. It must be said that as in several aspects of medical practice, there is not a general consensus among the experts regarding how much weight should be given to the various risk factors.

Genetics: It has been observed that the condition has the tendency to occur in families. For example, it has been observed that if a mother suffered from the condition, some of her daughters also may have gone on to suffer from the condition.

Personal History of Breast Cancer: A woman who has had cancer in one breast has an increased risk of developing a new cancer in the other breast or in another part of the same breast. This is different from a recurrence (return) of the first cancer.

Age at Childbirth: Studies have shown that women who happened to give birth to their first child at an older age or who have never given birth run the risk of developing the condition.

Contraceptive Pill: Women who take the contraceptive pill have been observed to tend to develop breast cancer as compared to women who are not on the pill.

Being overweight or obese: Being overweight or obese has been found to increase the risk of breast cancer, especially after menopause.

Alcohol: the use of alcohol increases the risk in the development of various cancers, including breast cancer. The rule seems to be the more alcohol one drinks the greater the risk of cancer.

Breastfeeding: Some studies suggest that breastfeeding may slightly lower breast cancer risk, especially if breastfeeding is continued for a period of about eighteen to twenty-four months. There are a few other risk factors in the literature which are not touched on here. Those interested in learning more may consult the relevant literature. For the sake of our current discussion, I consider the points already touched on to be sufficient.

DIAGNOSIS

Self-Examination: In breast cancer, self-examination by a woman if properly done can be an invaluable screening method. Health experts advise women to begin self-examining their breast by the age of twenty years. In this connection the experts recommend that women examine themselves about a week after the first day of their period, at a time when the breasts are no longer swollen and tender due to hormonal fluctuations. Any new changes should be reported to a doctor or a health professional, as the case may be. Of course, this recommendation can apply only to women living in areas where there is easy access to medical care. For women living in remote areas of our planet, like the remote African village where my eyes first saw the light of day, matters are not that straightforward.

What should a woman look out for on self-examining her breasts?

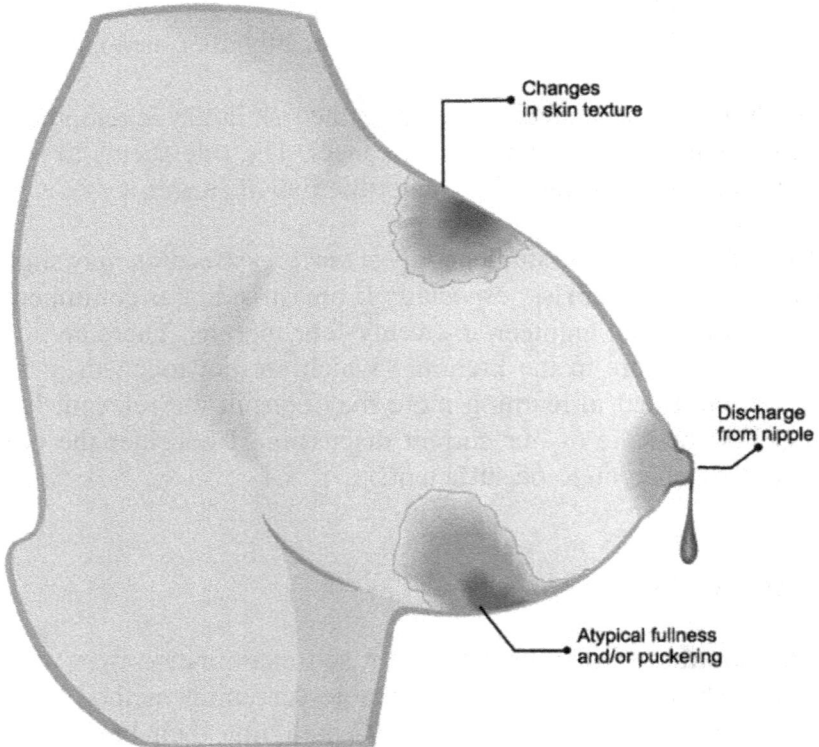

Breast self-exam:
visual inspection

Changes
in skin texture

Discharge
from nipple

Atypical fullness
and/or puckering

Changes in breast cancer

- Changes in the look or feel of the skin over the breast, especially if it looks dimpled, puckered or like orange peel.
- A lump, or a thickening or bumpy area in the breast or armpit, which is absent from the other breast or armpit.
- A discharge from the nipple that is new and which is not milk.

- More than the ordinary discomfort or pain in one breast, particularly if it refuses to go away after several days.
- Bleeding from the nipple.
- Any changes in the nipple position, like when it appears to be pulled up or pointing differently.
- A rash on or around the nipple.
- Moist red areas on the nipple that do not heal easily.
- A breast that feels warm to touch, much warmer than the other breast. It could be a sign of inflammatory breast cancer.

Clinical Breast Examination: Apart from self-examination, it is recommended that women above the age of twenty undergo clinical breast examination once a year through a nurse, a family doctor or a gynaecologist as the case may be. (In this case also it is a matter of access to corresponding medical care.)

Mammogram: This can be described as a breast x-ray. It is regarded as the gold standard for breast cancer screening and early detection. In some advanced societies, it is recommended that women above the age of 40 years have an annual mammogram. Mammograms are credited to help detect 85 to 90 per cent of all breast cancers, even those that are too small to be felt during manual examination.

TREATMENT

Treatment for breast cancer is based on the general principles of cancer treatment outlined above.

Surgery: Surgery could be in the form of:

- **Lumpectomy:** which involves the removal of the tumour and a small amount of normal tissue around it.
- **Partial mastectomy**: removal of the part of the breast that has cancer and some normal tissue around it.
- **Total mastectomy:** this type of surgery is resorted to in an advanced stage of cancer, when cancer might already have spread

to other parts of the body. This involves complete removal of the breast and surrounding tissue, including lymph nodes.

Surgery could be followed by one or more of the following:

- **Radiation therapy**
- **Chemotherapy**
- **Hormone therapy**. It is believed that hormones produced in the body sustain the growth of cancer cells. The aim of hormone therapy is to block the effect of such hormones on the growth of the breast cancer cells.

CHAPTER 31

Cervical Cancer

C ERVICAL CANCER is cancer affecting the cervix or the neck of the uterus (womb).

CAUSES

Medical science cannot exactly pinpoint the cause of cervical cancer. However, it has been established that the condition is strongly associated with Human Papilloma Virus (HPV)

RISK FACTORS

There are several risk factors. This book will touch on some of them. What I said about breast cancer is also true here—those wanting to know more are advised to read the relevant literature.

Human Papilloma Virus: HPV infection is one of the most significant risk factors in cervical cancer. This does not imply that every HPV infection will lead to cervical cancer. There are said to be approximately forty-six different kinds of HPV. Of the number only a few lead to the development of cancer. (As you may recall, one strain of the virus causes genital warts.)

Sexual behaviour: As we saw above, the Human Papilloma Virus is sexually transmitted.

The development of cervical cancer is thus strongly correlated with sexual behaviour. It is generally agreed that a woman has a higher risk of developing cervical cancer if she:
• Has had multiple sexual partners.
• Began having sexual relations early. By that the literature generally speaks of sexual contact before the age of 18 years. ·
• Has sex with partners who themselves have many partners.

The risks associated with sexual behaviour come down, in the end, to the risk of HPV infection. In this connection emphasis needs to be placed on the number of sexual partners. The more sexual partners one has, the more likely is the chance of contracting an HPV infection which could eventually develop into cervical cancer. For example, a 17-year-old who stays with the same faithful partner, who in turn remains faithful to her, is less likely to be infected by HPV and go on to develop cervical cancer, than the case of a 20-year-old who has multiple partners who, on their part, also boast of multiple partners.

Smoking: Women who smoke are about twice as likely to develop cervical cancer as women who do not. The more a woman smokes—and the longer she has been smoking—the greater the risk.

Weakened immune system: As I mentioned earlier, a weakened immune system generally impairs the body's ability to fight infections and other diseases, including cancer, in this case cervical cancer.

SYMPTOMS

In its early stage, cervical cancer may not cause noticeable signs or symptoms. Later signs of cervical cancer include:

- **Abnormal genital bleeding**. Genital bleeding is however not unique for cervical cancer—other conditions could be present with similar symptoms.
- **Unusual vaginal discharge**. It may be foul smelling, watery, thick, or contain mucus. This is also not unique for cervical cancer.
- **Pelvic pain.** This can be mild or severe and can range from a dull ache to a sharp pain. It can persist for hours.
- **Pain and or bleeding after or during sexual intercourse**.

DIAGNOSIS

- Clinical Examination.
- Smear test (Pap smear). This involves scraping cells off the cervix and smearing them onto a glass slide and analysing them under a microscope for abnormality.
- Coloscopy. In coloscopy, a device known as a coloscope is used to view and examine the surface of the cervix for signs of abnormality. This also allows for the taking of a biopsy for further examination.

TREATMENT

In this case the general principles of cancer therapy also apply.

SURGERY

This may involve the following:
- **Conization**: This procedure involves the removal of a cone-shaped piece of tissue from the cervix and cervical canal.
- **Cryosurgery**: In this type of treatment an instrument is used to freeze and destroy the cancer cells (abnormal tissue).
- **Laser Surgery**: In this procedure a laser beam, a narrow beam of intense light, is applied like a knife to cut out and remove the tumour.

The above three methods are only used in cases where the tumour is discovered in the very early stages, at a time when it is confined only to the cervix.

- **Hysterectomy**: The term stands for the complete removal of the womb. This method is applied in cases where the cancer has already reached an advanced stage. There are two forms of the procedure:
    - **Total hysterectomy**, which involves the removal of the uterus and cervix
    - **Radical hysterectomy**, which involves not only the removal of the entire womb, but also the ovaries, fallopian tubes and surrounding lymph nodes.

CHAPTER 32

Cancer of the Womb
(Endometrial Cancer)

IN THE PREVIOUS section we dealt with cancer of the cervix. As we learnt, this is cancer that affects the neck of the womb. I will now move on to consider cancer of the womb proper. The hollow of the womb is lined by a layer of cells known as endometrium. As in the case of almost every cell of the body, cancer cells can develop from the cells of the endometrium. Endometrial cancer is the fourth most common cancer that affects women, after breast, lung and colon cancer. It becomes more common after menopause.

RISK FACTORS

As in cervical cancer, it is not exactly known what causes cancer of the womb. Certain factors have however been observed to increase the risk. These include the following:

- Women who have never been pregnant: Studies have shown that women who have never given birth have a higher risk of developing the condition. Conversely the risk is lower in women who have had children.
- Obesity: Overweight or obese women are generally more likely to develop womb cancer than women of a normal weight.

- Age: Cancer of the womb becomes more common after menopause.
- Alcohol: Some studies have shown that women who drink considerable amounts of alcohol regularly have an increased risk of womb cancer compared to women who do not drink at all.

DIAGNOSIS

- **Clinical examination**.
  Depending on the medical facilities available, the clinical examination could be followed by one or more of the tests outlined below:
- **Biopsy**: As we saw earlier on, this involves the removal of tissue from the womb for further examination.
- **Hysteroscopy**: Where available, a device known as a hysteroscope can be used to view the inside of the womb. In the process a biopsy is taken.
- **Ultrasound scan**.

THERAPY

Surgery is one of the effective options to treat cancer of the womb. There are different types of surgeries that may be used, depending on the patient's condition. One of the common surgical procedures is total hysterectomy. This involves the complete removal of the womb, including the cervix. Depending on the type of cancer, the stage of disease and the extent to which the cancer has spread, radiotherapy, hormone therapy and chemotherapy may also be resorted to, either in isolation or in combination with surgery.

CHAPTER 33
Lung Cancer

⎯

LIKE ALL ORGANS of the body, the lung cells can also develop into cancer cells. The lung happens also to be a common site for the spread of cancers that have developed elsewhere in the body.

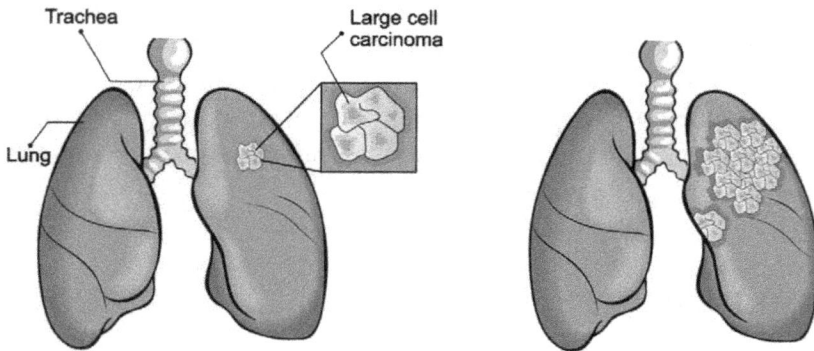

Lung Cancer

RISK FACTORS

- **Smoking**: The main risk factor in the development of lung cancer is cigarette smoking. It is true that there are instances when non-smokers have developed lung cancer. In the overwhelming number of cases (about nine out of ten), however, smokers are affected, whereas cigarette smokers are more at risk compared to pipe and cigar smokers.

- **Passive smoking:** Passive smoking, that is, the inhalation or breathing in of tobacco/ cigarette smoke coming from other smokers, does increase the risk for the development of lung cancer, though this risk is much less than that for the active smoker. In this connection, it is very encouraging that in several countries laws have been put in place to ban smoking in public places. It is hoped that those countries that have not done so, will sooner rather than later follow suit.

Other factors that increase the risk for the development of lung cancer are:

- **Asbetos**. Asbestos is the name given to a group of minerals that occur naturally in the environment as bundles of fibres. Individuals exposed to such fibres have an increased risk of developing lung cancer.
- **Radon gas.** Radon is a naturally occurring gas that seeps out of the ground in certain places. Studies have shown that individuals who are exposed to high concentrations of radon for a considerable period of time have an increased risk of developing lung cancer.
- **Air pollution**. Air pollution from vehicles, industry, and power plants, etc., is thought to have a small but significant increase in a person's lung cancer risk.

SYMPTOMS

As in the case of several forms of cancer, lung cancer may not cause any symptoms in the initial stages. As the disease advances, the following symptoms may become apparent:
- Shortness of breath
- Persistent coughing
- Coughing up blood
- Wheezing
- Chest pain

It must be said that the above symptoms are not exclusive for lung cancer. For example, lung tuberculosis can also lead to persistent coughing, and coughing of blood. Similarly, asthma may lead to shortness of breath and wheezing. If, however, the symptoms appear in a person who has a long history of smoking and are accompanied by the other general cancer symptoms touched on earlier, one should suspect lung cancer.

DIAGNOSIS

- **Clinical examination**
- **X-ray**: Chest x-ray is the most common first diagnostic step.
- **CT-scan**: This can help not only to establish the primary tumour, but also to reveal the spread of the disease.
- **MRI-scan**.
- **Sputum cytology**: This involves the examination of the sputum of the affected person for evidence of cancer cells.
- **Bronchoscopy**: Where available, a device known as a bronchoscope is used to view the airways for signs of cancer. In the process a biopsy is taken for further examination.

TREATMENT

As in the majority of cancers, treatment involves surgery, radiotherapy and chemotherapy. These may be offered alone or in combination, depending on the type of cancer in question (there are two main types, non-small-cell lung cancer or small-cell lung cancer), how well the patient is and also the extent to which cancer has spread to other parts of the body.

CHAPTER 34

Prostate Cancer

EARLIER I dealt with benign prostate hyperplasia (BPH) and the symptoms associated with it. I will now turn my attention to cancer of the prostate gland.

CAUSES

Medical science cannot exactly pinpoint the causes.

RISK FACTORS

The following are some of the common risk factors linked with the condition:
- **Age**: It has been said that prostate cancer is a disease of old age. Men aged below 50 years have a low risk of developing the condition. The risk increases considerably after that age. It's estimated that around 80% of men in their 80s will have prostate cancer.
- **Ethnic background**: It has been observed that men of African descent are more likely to be affected than men of European and Asian descent.

- **Family history**: It has also been observed that men whose close relatives—father, brother, grandfather—have had the condition are slightly more likely to develop it themselves.

SYMPTOMS

The symptoms of prostate cancer can be similar to that occurring in BPH. They may include the following:
- Urinating frequently.
- Difficult or painful urination or ejaculation.
- Delay or hesitancy before urinating.
- A feeling that the bladder has not completely emptied.
- Blood in urine or semen.
- Disturbed sleep because of the need to empty the bladder at night.

DIAGNOSIS

Prostate-specific antigen (PSA) test: The main test for prostate cancer is the PSA test. PSA is a substance found in the blood of men. A rise of PSA above a certain value is a possible indication of prostate cancer. There is some current concern, however, about the accuracy of the PSA test and its usefulness. Some studies have shown that
- Up to 20% of men who do have prostate cancer will not have a raised PSA level;
- Over 65% of men with a raised PSA level will not have cancer since PSA levels tend to rise in all men as they get older.

Clinical Examination: The next step in confirming a diagnosis of prostate cancer is by way of clinical examination, specifically, by way of digital rectal examination (DRE). This involves the examiner inserting a finger in the rectum (back passage). The rectum is close to the prostate gland, a fact which enables the examiner to feel it. Usually the surface of the gland feels smooth to touch. Prostate cancer can cause the gland to become hard and bumpy. An experienced examiner will notice the difference and suspect cancer.

Biopsy: Cancer is usually established by taking a piece of tissue and examining it under the microscope.

Ultra Sound: Where available, the prostate gland can be examined with a type of ultrasound called transrectal ultrasonography. This is inserted into the rectum (back passage) to the nearby prostate.

MRI-Scan: MRI scans can create a clear picture of the prostate gland.

CT Scan: Tumors can better be seen with CT-Scans than with an ordinary X-ray

TREATMENT

If diagnosed early, treatment can be quite successful. The key decision in prostate cancer is whether or not to treat at all. In many older men, the cancer progresses so slowly that surgery and other treatments may cause more harm than good. However, for those whose cancer is more aggressive, either already spreading or liable to spread beyond the prostate, surgery is usually the first option. Surgery involves the removal of the gland (prostatectomy) together with surrounding lymph nodes.

Surgery may lead to nerve damage, which in turn may lead to erection as well as urinary problems.

CHAPTER 35

Skin Cancer

The main cause of skin cancer is overexposure to the sun's harmful ultraviolet (UV) rays.

OTHER RISK FACTORS

People with fair skin: Statistics have shown that the light-skinned individual is more vulnerable to develop the condition. It must be stressed that having a light skin alone is not an all-determining factor. What may have been observed to aggravate the situation is an over-exposure of the skin to ultraviolet rays, such as occurs during sunbathing.

Family history: People with a family history of melanoma have roughly double the risk of developing the disease compared to people without a family history

TYPES OF SKIN CANCER

BASAL CELL CARCINOMA: This is the most common type of skin cancer. It affects the basal cells. These are found within the top layer of skin. It is a slow-growing cancer and does not usually metastasize or spread to other parts of the body. Basal cell carcinoma affects all sun exposed areas of the body

Symptoms:
It may appear as a small painless lump, brownish-grey in colour. It may develop a central depression with rolled edges.

SQUAMOUS CELL CARCINOMA: This type of skin cancer usually affects the face.

Symptoms:
The main symptom is an area of thickened, scaly skin. This may develop into a painless, hard lump, reddish brown in colour with an irregular edge. The lump could develop into an ulcer which won't heal.

The above-named types of skin cancer are known as non-melanoma skin cancer to differentiate them from melanoma.

MELANOMA SKIN CANCER: Melanoma of the skin is related to the common mole. It is the most aggressive form of skin cancer and can occur anywhere on the body. It affects the melanin cells, the cells which produce the skin's colouring. If not identified and treated early, it can spread to affect the liver, lungs or brain.

Symptoms:
The main symptoms are: a quick-growing, irregular, dark-coloured spot on previously normal skin or on an existing mole that changes size, colour, develops irregular edges, bleeds, itches, crusts or reddens.

DIAGNOSIS

- **Clinical examination**: The condition might be suspected as a result of the changes outlined above.
- **Biopsy**: Any potential melanoma requires a surgical biopsy, also known as excisional biopsy, in which the entire growth is removed. The sample is then studied under a microscope to determine whether cancer cells are present.

TREATMENT OF SKIN CANCER

NON-MELANOMA:

- **Surgery**: Non-melanoma skin cancers are usually treated by a common operation to simply cut out the affected area under local anaesthetic.
- **Cryosurgery**: Another method used on smaller cancers is cryosurgery, in which liquid nitrogen is applied to the tumour to freeze it and kill the cells. The tumour will simply wither and drop off once warmed up.
- **Photodynamic therapy**: A so-called 'photodynamic therapy' is applied to treat some cases of basal cell carcinoma. This involves the use of a cream to sensitise the tumour. It is then exposed to high intensities of light to destroy it.

MELANOMA:

Treatment for melanoma depends on the extent of the disease, the patient's age and general health, and other factors.

Apart from the three general forms of cancer treatment outlined earlier, namely surgery, radiation therapy, chemotherapy, a fourth type, biological therapy, may be applied. Biological therapy, making use of special proteins known as interferon, is resorted to especially in cases where cancer has spread to other parts of the body or in patients where there is a high risk of the cancer returning. Interferon acts to stimulate immune cells into attacking melanoma cells more aggressively.

PART 7

MENTAL HEALTH ISSUES

CHAPTER 36

Anxiety & Depression

$\sim$

ANXIETY is a troubled state of mind characterised by uneasiness and apprehension—an almost permanent feeling of fear, worry as well as a feeling of being weighed down with care and concern, especially for the future.

Everyone experiences a certain degree of anxiety at some stage in life. I have in mind the football player or fan whose team is engaged in a penalty shootout to decide the outcome of a crucial match. The heart as a result of the tense situation could start racing, the muscles could begin shaking involuntarily, sweat could break out to soak our clothes, etc. Our team could end up losing the match. That could lead, in the short term, to disappointment, even bitter disappointment. That in turn could even lead to a sleepless night. That is a natural human reaction to a distressing situation.

The problem begins when anxiety, as it were, becomes an almost permanent guest in our home—when we begin to develop an excessive, uncontrollable and often irrational worry about everyday things, disproportionate to the actual source of worry. At this stage medical science speaks of generalised anxiety disorder.

CAUSES

The following are some of the factors identified by medical science as possible causes of anxiety.

- **Genes**: The fact that some tend to be more anxious than others has led medical science to conclude that it could have something to do with the genes we inherited from our parents. I personally take this explanation with a pinch of salt. I am inclined to think that an increased tendency to become anxious has more to do with our upbringing than our genes. Parents who tend to be anxious about many things may bring up their children in such a way as to impart that tendency on them.
- **Circumstances**: Our circumstances may lead to anxiety. For example, the threat of job loss, of deportation, of repossession of our homes, etc., may lead to anxiety.
- **Drugs**: The so-called recreational drugs like amphetamines, lysergic acid diethylamide, abbreviated LSD or ecstasy can lead to anxiety after their so-called "pleasurable effects" have subsided.

SYMPTOMS

The example about the penalty shootout touched on some of the symptoms associated with anxiety. These include the following:
- Feeling worried all the time
- Tiredness
- Irritability
- Sleep disturbance
- Difficulty concentrating
- Racing heartbeat
- Sweating
- Muscle tension and pains
- Shaking
- Feeling dizzy or faint

PANIC

This is a special form of anxiety and involves sudden and unexpected episodes of intense anxiety. Panic attacks share some of the symptoms of anxiety, e.g. accelerated heart rate, shaking, sweating, feeling dizzy, etc., though the said symptoms are experienced more intensely by the affected person.

DEPRESSION

Anxiety and depression are related in the sense that anxiety leads to depression. Anxiety is short-lived. Anxiety, should it persist for a long while, ends up in depression.

The state of mind of the depressed person is characterized among other things by feelings of sadness, gloom, despair, low self-esteem, self-reproach and discouragement. The following are some of the life events that can lead to depression:

- **Bereavement**: Death of a family member, friend, or pet. Indeed, the death of a pet can lead to depression in some individuals.
- **Breakdown of relationships:** This can lead to depression not only in the affected individuals themselves but may also lead to depression in their children.
- **Birth of a child (postnatal depression):** What is usually regarded as a happy event can, unfortunately, lead to depression in some mothers.
- **Stressful situations**: Poverty, homelessness, job loss, violence in the family, constant relationship problems, etc., could also lead to depression.

FORMS OF DEPRESSION

Depression can come in various forms:

- **Major Depression**: Also known as unipolar depression, major depression could be intense and short-lived.
- **Dysthymia**: Also known as chronic depression; this type of depression, though less severe, is long-lasting.

- **Bipolar Disorder**: Bipolar disorder is characterized by periods of major depression alternating or combined with periods of mania. In mania the affected person experiences abnormally high moods and extreme bursts of unusual activity or energy. So, a person suffering a bipolar disorder feels down one day and extremely happy the next.

SYMPTOMS

A person suffering from depression may lose interest in life, a situation that could in turn lead to suicidal thoughts, attempts or in the worst case scenario, suicide.

Other symptoms are:

- Feeling of worthlessness
- Feeling of hopelessness
- Feeling of pessimism
- Feeling of guilt
- Finding it harder to make decisions
- Not coping with things that used to be manageable
- Exhaustion
- Feeling restless and agitated
- Loss of appetite and weight
- Sleeping difficulty

In short, as far as the depressed person is concerned, everything is gloom, gloom, gloom. He or she, as it were, considers him or herself as entrapped in a dark tunnel or locked up in an abyss of thick darkness. Whereas others in such a situation may discern a ray of light in the thick cloud of darkness, the depressed individual sees nothing but darkness, darkness, darkness.

DRUG TREATMENT OF ANXIETY AND DEPRESSION

Following are some of the anti-depressants in use:
- Selective serotonin re-uptake inhibitors (SSRIs)—an example of this group of medication is Citalopram.
- Atypical antidepressants: These are described as atypical antidepressants because medical science does not understand exactly the mechanisms of their action. An example is Mirtazapine.
- Tricyclic antidepressants (TCAs): An example of this group is amitriptyline.
- Monoamine oxidase inhibitors (MAOIs): An example is Phenelzine (Nardil)

The antidepressants listed above have one thing in common: they all have considerable side effects—side effects that could be so severe as to lead to the interruption of therapy.

Plant-based drugs: Apart from the above-named group of medication, a few plant-based drugs are used in the treatment of anxiety and depression. An example is St. John's wort (*Hypericum perforatum*) which is popular, especially in Germany.

NON-DRUG THERAPY

Apart from medication, *psychotherapy* is employed in the treatment of anxiety and depression. One may want to know what the term stands for. It is a branch of psychiatry which employs dialogue and a variety of communication techniques with the aim of treating individuals suffering from mental and emotional disorders. In the treatment of depression, psychotherapy aims at helping the patient develop new ways to cope with challenges in life, and to identify and understand more about depression and how to avoid it in the future.

Psychotherapy is also known as "talk" therapy. During the talking sessions that may take place in groups or on a one-to-one basis, the skilled psychotherapist may use one or more of the following strategies:

- Pinpoint the life problems that contributed to the patient's depression, and help him or her to understand which aspects of those problems he or she may be able to solve or improve.
- Identify negative or distorted thinking patterns that contribute to feelings of hopelessness and helplessness that accompany depression.
- Explore other learned thoughts and behaviours that create problems and contribute to depression.
- Help people regain a sense of control and pleasure in life.

CHAPTER 37

Good Night And Sleep Well

INSOMNIA is the chronic inability to fall asleep or remain asleep for an adequate length of time. The brain requires regular and adequate sleep to regenerate itself so that it may continue to function properly. This inevitably leads to the question: how much sleep is adequate for the human being? A new-born usually sleeps between 16 and 19 hours per day; this reduces to about 12 hours by the age of 5 years. For most adults, 7 to 8 hours a night appears to be the best amount of sleep, although the amount ranges from 5 hours to 10 hours of sleep each day depending on the individual.

Unfortunately in the modern world, due to various reasons—domestic and work demands, social responsibilities, unhealthy lifestyles (some sit before the computer and play games deep, deep into the night!)—it is becoming increasingly difficult for some individuals to get adequate sleep.

ON THE USE OF SLEEPING TABLETS

For those who suffer from chronic sleeplessness, sleeping tablets can be an answer. It is important, though, that therapy aims first at the root cause of the problem rather than the symptoms. Lack of sleep could be secondary to depression which in turn could be a result of burdens on the mind that need to be alleviated.

After several weeks of use, sleeping pills begin to lose their efficacy, which may call for an increase in dosage to achieve the desired effect. In the end one could become addicted to them.

Before you consider buying over-the-counter sleeping tablets or asking your doctor to prescribe those requiring a doctor's prescription, you may consider the following tips aimed at promoting a more restful and effective sleep:

- It is important to have a good bedtime routine. As far as possible try to go to bed at about the same time every night. This should be the case whether one is tired or not.
- The bedroom should have the right environment, not too hot or cold; not too noisy.
- One should undertake some moderate exercise every day—swimming, walking or jogging. This is particularly important for people who have a sedentary lifestyle or who are not engaged in strenuous physical work.
- It is important to avoid any stimulant drinks, especially coffee several hours before the fall of darkness.
- One should also avoid eating too much late into the night.
- Some have reported that drinking a cup or two of milk or chamomile tea before retiring to bed has a favourable influence on sleep.
- Listening to music, restful classical music, is also reported to help induce sleep.

Good night and sleep well, dear reader!

www.ingramcontent.com/pod-product-compliance
Lightning Source LLC
Chambersburg PA
CBHW031513270326
41930CB00006B/389